NATURE'S
DIRTY
NEEDLE

WHAT YOU NEED TO KNOW ABOUT
CHRONIC LYME DISEASE AND HOW TO
GET THE HELP TO FEEL BETTER

MARA WILLIAMS
RN, MSN, ANP-BC

D1445103

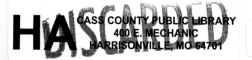

NATURE'S DIRTY NEEDLE

WHAT YOU NEED TO KNOW ABOUT CHRONIC LYME DISEASE AND HOW TO GET THE HELP TO FEEL BETTER

MARA WILLIAMS

Copyright© 2011
ISBN 978-1-937445-09-6
Library of Congress Control Number: 2011936501

Published by Bush Street Press
237 Kearny Street, #174
San Francisco, CA 94108
415-413-0785

DEDICATION

I DEDICATE THIS BOOK TO all of you who have been ill for many years and have struggled on a daily basis to get help and feel better against difficult odds.

TABLE OF CONTENTS

FOREWORD

I HAVE HAD THE PLEASURE and privilege of working with Mara Williams for the past two years.

I know that she is dedicated to helping the thousands of unfortunate patients who have contracted Lyme disease and its co-infections, and that she is motivated by both a deep desire to heal all of those who come to her for medical treatment, and by her personal struggle to help her own daughter, who has come down with an unusually severe case of Lyme disease.

All of us who work with Lyme disease have experienced the profound frustration of trying to swim against the current of medical beliefs that surround this illness. It is a disease embroiled in controversy. There are many well-meaning physicians who are unaware of how prevalent and devastating it can be. A large medical contingent called the Infectious Disease Society of America (IDSA) has been highly visible and vocal in their belief that there is no such thing as chronic Lyme disease. They admit that there is something which they call Post-Lyme Syndrome, but they have no specific treatment to offer for it. Unfortunately, their influence on other physicians has been considerable. The CDC does not recognize the existence of chronic Lyme disease, so there is no ongoing research. This leaves us somewhere between a rock and hard place.

Our tests are nowhere near as accurate as we need them to be, and as Mara reiterates, the only test worth doing is the IGenex Western Blot panels. Many patients are under the impression that they have been tested adequately for Lyme disease when they have only had a "screening" test for Lyme. That test, which is an antibody test and not a Western Blot test, is virtually useless in the identification of individuals who have Lyme disease, and it allows a physician to suggest to a patient that they have been accurately tested for Lyme disease, when in fact, they have not. This allows the disease to go undiagnosed for years, which is a common thread in the stories that Mara relates in her book. When Lyme disease goes untreated for more than a year, it can become a living nightmare. It is also a travesty. I find myself apologizing every single day for the oversights of my colleagues in both the diagnosis and treatment of this disease. Untreated patients and their families can be devastated by this illness.

Fortunately, there is another medical association, the International Lyme and Associated Disease Society (ILADS), who does recognize the extent and importance of identifying and treating patients with chronic Lyme disease. They have pioneered treatment programs and are making every effort to educate physicians and patients in the understanding of this problem.

In this book, Mara uses the real-life stories of her patients to bring home the poignancy of this disease. She emphasizes the vast parade of symptoms which make diagnosis so complicated, allowing us to call

Lyme disease "the great masquerader." She emphasizes the difficulties in diagnosis and the corresponding difficulties in treatment.

One of the most important take-home messages of this book is to ask all of you, or your loved ones, to *please* think about or consider the possibility of Lyme disease when you have been truly ill, and your doctors have not provided a clear diagnosis, or an effective treatment. It is much more common than you have been led to believe. It *can* be treated, especially when it is diagnosed early.

When patients are in the throes of severe Lyme disease, they may have nowhere to go and nowhere to turn. Since many physicians and hospitals believe that Lyme disease is a trivial or non-existent problem, the usual places that patients turn in times of need are of little help. When the co-infections Bartonella and Babesia kick in and patients feel anxious, panicky, and depressed to the point of despair, simple antidepressants are not sufficient. They need a safe haven, where their illness will be understood, their suffering appreciated, and appropriate treatment can be provided. Mara's vision of Inanna House is sorely needed and would be a breath of fresh air for those in need. Please read her book and learn more.

Neil Nathan, MD
Author of *On Hope and Healing: For Those Who Have Fallen Through the Medical Cracks*
Gordon Medical Associates
Santa Rosa, California

INTRODUCTION

AS A NURSE PRACTITIONER, I have been blessed to work with some amazing and courageous physicians who practice "out of the box" medicine. Using herbals, neutraceuticals, as well as pharmaceuticals to offer the best of both natural and allopathic ways of health care, this group of providers gives their best to help people discover the root cause of their problem and get well. They listen and spend the time to understand what is going on with a person, what their story is telling them, and the clinical picture being presented. In the past three years, I have focused on Chronic Lyme Disease (CLD) and other illnesses that cause chronic and debilitating illness. Then a little over a year ago, I realized that my daughter, Amanda, was very sick with CLD. It was a stunning moment. Fortunately, I work with providers who can help her as I had to assume the role of mother once again. What our family has endured when it becomes necessary to interact with the current health care system is a horror story. It is this experience that has compelled me to write this book. Amanda's story and the others in this book must be told. Hopefully, this will lead to greater awareness of the worldwide issue of CLD, the politics around it, and how to get help and feel better.

1: ENTER THE LYME WARS

THE CURRENT HEALTH CARE SYSTEM is broken and is beyond repair. It is driven by profit and controlled by the insurance and pharmaceutical industries. Millions of people are marginalized, forgotten, and left without the ability to live productive lives. Approximately one-third of the United States population is without health insurance and, yet, we as a nation pay over $6,000 per person to sustain the current system, which is geared toward the middle-aged man in crisis. It is left up to families to care for those who are abandoned by the system, further depleting resources and creating a huge impact on the economy.

There is an epidemic sweeping the world that is denied by the Western Health Care System: Chronic Lyme Disease and its co-infections that are carried by ticks and other insects, including mosquitos, fleas, biting flies, and mites. These diseases do not fit into a neat package. They are complex and challenging to treat. This complexity demands that each individual be considered separately- as an individual. On the average, someone with CLD sees 30 providers before finding one that understands their problems. I chose to begin with this story as Talia is healthy and cured. I wanted the first message to be one of hope.

TALIA'S STORY - IN HER OWN WORDS

"It was 2004, and I had started telling people I had a "blood infection." It was the only way I could describe what I felt was going on in my body. I'd felt sick for some time, and it was affecting everything in my life. I couldn't get any help from doctors, but I knew something was terribly wrong. I was having recurring bouts with what felt like a mild flu. I never threw up or got high fevers when these bouts hit, but would feel awful and mostly need to stay in bed and sleep.

It was late in that year that someone I knew who had Lyme disease listened to my list of ailments and said, "I think you better get checked for Lyme. That stuff sounds awfully familiar." She referred me to IGenex lab to get tested. I came back positive for Lyme and Babesia. What was amazing and wonderful was to hear the list of symptoms associated with these, and related bugs, and suddenly have an explanation for ALL the strange and horrible stuff I'd been experiencing for years. There was stuff on that symptom list that I'd worried about, asked doctors about, and never had any explanation given. It went well beyond the recurring bouts of flu. There was the numbness in my hands, the night sweats, the mental confusion/haze, the irritable bladder, agoraphobia, joint pain, hormonal problems that had been attributed to me "getting older" (at age 30!) and more.

The diagnosis came as a tremendous relief. Tracking the symptoms, I realized I probably had the Lyme infection for at least five years at that time, possibly more. As I did research online one day, I found pictures of the EM, or "bull's-eye" rash. I saw a few images before one made me nearly fall out of my chair. The particular shape and form of that image was not unfamiliar to me! I'd had that same rash on my leg. I could not place exactly when, but I remembered it distinctly as soon as I saw the image. It had been about eight inches long, up from about my ankle. I'd thought at the time it was a spider bite that I was having a strange reaction to. Since the rash was not painful or itchy, I didn't give it another thought. Not until seeing the image online all those years later, did it gain any significance.

I was very lucky. I was treated for my illness at a great private clinic by a wonderful physician's assistant who had made himself an expert in treating Lyme disease. I got the best care and was symptom free and "cured" in two years. That is a very fast course of healing for this disease, especially compared to the agony many patients go through. I've heard of people who have drip IVs for years at a time, one woman who had her gall bladder removed, and courses of "treatment" that go on for ten years or more without helping.

My treatment began with Mepron, an intense pharmaceutical drug that is an antimicrobial, used to treat Babesia. My doctor explained to me that it was important to go after the Babesia first as it somehow "hides" and "protects" the Lyme bug. He described a process that sounded a bit like peeling an onion. If we didn't get the outer layer first, our efforts to treat anything underneath would be ineffective. I understood then why people spent years and years on antibiotics and never got better. Luckily, my treatment

was different. I took Mepron for about eight months
before all my symptoms were gone. It was powerful
stuff, and it made me feel much worse before I felt
better. That was how I knew it was working. Again, my
doctor explained things to me. He said that as the bug
is killed off, it releases its neurotoxins. This "die-off" as
the medicine is working then makes you feel worse for
a time as your system is flooded with toxins. The
important thing is to hang in there through it, making
sure to keep your body flushing itself out well. I was
also taking Azithromycin at the same time. With all
these heavy antibiotics, I also took heavy doses of
probiotics the whole time. After several months, I was
truly getting some relief from what had been some of
my worst symptoms. For one thing, the mental
confusion cleared up tremendously. I started to feel a
little more like myself for the first time in many long
years. I was treated for several other "co-infections"
next, using a combination of various antibiotics, as
well as homeopathic and herbal treatments. None of it
was as tough as the Mepron had been. I was already
feeling worlds better. My treatment ended with finally
addressing the Lyme bug. I had three or four months of
Bicillin injections, twice a week. They were painful
injections, but I didn't mind. The cure was much better
than the alternative of suffering with illness! And I
knew that I was in the home stretch. I finished that
course of antibiotics pretty tired. It had been two years.
I told my doctor I'd had enough. I felt I was feeling the
effects of the antibiotic more than the bug. We were
done. In an amazingly short period of time, I was
through it.

It boggles my mind and makes me furious that people are not getting diagnosed and treated, so they can be well again. Then I hear of the lucky ones who get diagnosed but the treatments are ineffectual and sometimes absurd. Then there are the sad cases in which the person continues undiagnosed. I even had a friend who suffered from seizures suddenly in her thirties. At first, doctors thought she had MS. I remember crying when I heard that news. Then they found it was not MS. They said she just had developed seizures with no explanation. She did have brain lesions that they couldn't explain, but they weren't dwelling on that. Her description of her symptoms reminded me of those described by author Amy Tan, who has Lyme disease and writes about it. I suggested my friend get tested and sent her to IGenex. She came back positive. But her doctor disputed the results, telling her she did not have Lyme, based on a spinal tap they'd done. She goes un-treated to this day and lives on heavy doses of anti-seizure medication.

For my part, I have been able to live a pain-free, physically active, alert, healthy life. I finished treatment and with the O.K. of my doctor, began trying to have the child I'd always wanted. I was pregnant quickly, and my son was born, as healthy as can be. I went back to grad school and earned my master's degree in psychology. I am able to take part in the joys of life, and that is quite a blessing. It is one I know, in my bones, everyone has a right to, and everyone has the ability to reach. There is very good medicine for treating these diseases; it just has to be done right. The tragic thing, to me, is that there are so few doctors out there who know how to do it right. But

there is a right way. There is a path out of the pain and
confusion. I have walked it. I hope that in some way, I
may now reach my hand out to help others to do the
same."

Talia has become an advocate for others now that
she has the energy to reach out in her community. She
has a passion for increasing awareness and to prevent
the suffering that these infections cause, especially
with children who are being misdiagnosed.

2: WHAT IS CHRONIC LYME DISEASE?

THE CENTER FOR DISEASE CONTROL (CDC) criteria for Lyme disease misses 90% of Lyme infections.

Chronic Lyme Disease is a worldwide epidemic. It is the fastest growing and most prevalent insect-borne infection in the United States. Chronic Lyme Disease is a complex of multiple co-infections resulting from the bite of an infected tick. It can be transmitted from a person who has been bitten by an infected tick through blood transfusions, organ donation, across the placental barrier to a fetus, sexually, through body fluids, and possibly through breast milk. Dr. Joe Burrascano, an expert in the field, defines Chronic Lyme Disease as being ill with Lyme/Tick-borne diseases (TBD) for greater than one year. He says that after one year of illness, the immune system begins to break down. The longer a person is sick, the more secondary damage and dysregulation will occur, and the more difficult it is to control the infection. This means that other systems in the body, like the immune system, the hormonal system, and autonomic nervous system, stop functioning in a healthy way. The immune system becomes hypersensitive to the constant insult of the bugs, and it goes haywire and reacts to everything. When this happens, people with CLD become sensitive to everything, including chemical sensitivity and mold toxin. The liver stops working optimally, and the body has a difficult time clearing toxins, which increases the intensity of symptoms. This creates systemic inflammation and other symptoms, which makes everything worse for the ill person, and it also makes treating more complex and difficult.

About 65% of people bitten by a tick do not know it. When a tick bites, a series of events begins quickly. The makeup of the tick's saliva is connected to these events. As a tick bites, it goes through the outer layer of skin to reach the blood vessels below the surface. Then a cement-like substance is secreted that causes hardening around the bite site. This anchors the tick in place and also forms a barrier that prevents blood loss. This cement is similar to collagen and keratin, which are major components of the skin. Once completely engorged, the tick falls off. The cement core is left in place, still embedded in the skin. While feeding, the tick alternates between taking blood and releasing saliva, which enters the blood and surrounding tissues of its victim. The saliva contains a complex blend of pharmacologically active compounds designed to counteract immune defenses that occur once someone is bitten. These include an inflammation response and an immune response. This allows the Lyme bug to easily enter through the salivary glands of the tick, find unprotected sites in the victim's body, and grow. (*Healing Lyme.* Stephan Harrod Buhner, 2005, pp.24-26).

If you are bitten by a tick and are aware of the bite, it is critical to seek advice from a Lyme-literate provider. Many people go to the emergency room or their primary physician and are told it is nothing to be concerned with, or the doctor may prescribe seven to ten days of an antibiotic, the usual time for most bacterial infections. This is inadequate treatment. If you see a rash around the bite, especially a circular rash, like a bull's eye, then you definitely have been infected with Lyme. The only way to avoid chronic and long-term illness is with a course of antibiotics for one to three months, especially if you have any symptoms. Lyme disease and the co-infections do not clear the body on their own. Seeing a Lyme–literate provider will give you the peace of mind that you will get better. If you choose to see your own primary physician, then demand the appropriate course of antibiotics. If you do not advocate for yourself, it is a set-up for chronic and long-term problems.

Marion's story shows her tenaciousness in searching for an answer to her illness. She did not give up, despite being repeatedly told there was nothing wrong with her.

MARION'S STORY

When Marion was 32 and her daughter was 1 year old, she started noticing "a ringworm rash" on her forearm, a little circle. Then she got a flu that didn't go away. She couldn't shake it. She had a baby and worked as a teacher, so life was full. Marion was depressed and felt there was no reason to be. This feeling would go away and then come back, again and again. Things started happening that she couldn't control. Everything became jumbled, and she felt she was losing her mind. She saw 36 doctors altogether during that year, as she was going from one symptom to the other. There was a lupus butterfly across her face. She forgot how to read. Mornings were the worst, since she couldn't get out of bed due to exhaustion and stiffness. She would throw up in the morning. As the day went on, she felt better. Her husband would find her lying on the ground in the middle of the night, and she wouldn't remember what happened, but she realized she was having seizures. Doctors started to tell her it was in her head. She went to a therapist and cried. Marion saw a psychiatrist for four years after she became pregnant and lost one of twins she was carrying.

Finally, she started talking to others who had Lyme disease. A neighbour who was sick had enough strength to fight with the physicians. She wrote to UCB and asked for their help. Her daughter was 7 years old when she started acting differently—crying, being moody, and finding that numbers made no sense in class. Marion was in a PTA meeting when she heard about another child with Lyme. She had her daughter tested, and the results came back positive. The doctor believed no child could get Lyme and refused to treat her. This stance was in the literature!

By that time, Marion was getting bull's eye rashes regularly. She then heard of Paul Lavioe, MD, who was treating Lyme at UC. This was at a time when no one believed Lyme was on the West coast. Her husband was diagnosed with cardiomyopathy, and he went to see Dr. Lavioe, which cost over $750.00 in late 1990's. Her insurance ended up paying for the visit. He spent 6 hours with Marion and her husband. Her husband was told his heart was affected and that nothing would reverse the damage. But the doctor said he could cure Marion. She went to Dr. Lavoie for treatment after that visit. He told her to exercise to make the bugs become active. She took massive doses of antibiotics and then went off of them until symptoms returned, then went back on the drugs in a pulsing fashion. A local doctor treated her daughter during this time. It was a huge hurdle for Marion to tell the doctor her symptoms after being told it was all in her head. Her tests had come back negative previously, but the doctor did labs with the flare up, and the labs were finally positive. Marion started doing alternative therapies like acupuncture, massage, wheat grass twice a day, vitamins and minerals, Chinese herbs, and other therapies.

Marion believes she was infected for seven years before treatment. When her son was two, he got Lyme. Marion found a tick on him. She got a doctor in the Sonoma valley to give her son antibiotics. He did two series of six weeks of an antibiotic. After the treatment, her son felt well, with no more symptoms. Once Marion realized she had Lyme disease, she called the psychiatrist and told him of her diagnosis. He had felt all along that she was infected with something. Through all of her search for help, Marion felt like she had fallen in a hole and couldn't climb out. It was impossible to read. She was having seizures. She couldn't walk. It was impossible to be in the sun because she was so light sensitive. Marion was on antibiotics on and off for six years when she decided to go off them and she see how she did.

She still had cycles of feeling poorly, but she could function and exercise. Alternative therapies are ongoing. She still has fatigue and nausea once in a while. Both of her children are well now. Marion realized years ago that it is necessary to work with her emotional issues and heal them, as well as the infections. She attributes being well to this work. Her story also points to the need for an integrative approach to healing CLD.

3: THE BUGS

LYME

BORRELIA BURGDORFERI, THE LYME BACTERIA, is a Spirochete bacteria shaped like a cork screw. It is similar to Syphilis, which loves to burrow into many different tissues in the body, including nervous tissue, joint tissue, connective tissue, muscles, the heart, and the brain. There are over 300 different types of Lyme or Borrelia. Borrelia can change its form from the typical cork screw shape to a cystic form, and an intracellular form. It can hide, evading the immune system or go dormant. It can create a bio-film that covers it, allowing it to hide more efficiently.

With Lyme, there is usually a gradual onset of symptoms, which come and go in four-week cycles. These symptoms involve many systems and are migratory. There is joint involvement, afternoon fevers with flu-like symptoms, neurological symptoms that can mimic many other medical conditions like Multiple Sclerosis, Parkinson's disease, and ALS (Lou Gehrig's disease). Fatigue is profound. Muscle weakness, difficulty walking, and numbness and tingling in the arms and legs are common. Mood and cognitive problems are usually moderate. Sleep can be mildly disruptive. Pain can be moderate to severe, unilateral or one-sided, or wandering, achy, and generalized. Usually, Lyme is slow growing, but there are a few aggressive forms.

THE CO-INFECTIONS

Multiple co-infections exist along with Borrelia that causes CLD. These are nearly universal now as a single tick can carry as many as seven different infectious pathogens. Co-infections include bacteria, fungus, parasites, and viruses. Co-infections are almost always present, and their symptoms are more intense and vague. They make diagnostic testing less reliable, and people become more ill and difficult to treat. Some of the bacteria, parasites, yeasts, and viruses must be treated with different medicines than what is prescribed to treat Lyme. This is one of the reasons for "treatment-resistant" Lyme.

Bartonella is a bacteria with about 28 different sub-species, including Cat Scratch Fever. Gradual onset of initial illness is common. Symptoms can differ depending on which side of the country you live. On the West Coast, Bartonella causes a multitude of symptoms. The bottoms of the feet are painful, burning, and /or numb. Pain and swelling in the joints, specifically, and pain in general are common. These symptoms can migrate from joint to joint. The pain is severe. Lymph glands can swell. Gastrointestinal symptoms can be severe, including painful cramping, persistent nausea with vomiting, weight loss, bloating, diarrhea, and constipation. Headaches are severe and begin in the back of the head and travel to the front. Mood changes can also be severe, including depression, anxiety, and panic attacks. Changes in the white matter of the brain can show up on SPEC scan, and the changes correlate with these symptoms. Cognitive problems include brain fog, loss of concentration, and memory loss. Sleep can be significantly disrupted. Inflammation of the vascular system occurs, leading to possible blood clots and cardio-vascular issues. There is a rapid relapse of symptoms if treatment is ended too soon. Patients describe the pain in their joints as, "I feel like my hips are breaking."

Babesia is a parasite that burrows into the red blood cells and is typically found with Bartonella. Usually, there is an abrupt onset of symptoms with the initial illness, including severe, drenching sweats, especially at night. Fatigue, global headaches, air hunger or shortness of breath, an increased heart rate that is noticeable, heat and cold intolerance, cough, and hypercoagulability are hallmarks of Babesia. Pain is less severe than with other infections. Mood and cognitive symptoms are severe. Sleep is disruptive and frequent waking occurs. Since it is a parasite, typical Lyme treatment produces no response. Babesia infections can intensify Lyme symptoms. Severe depression with suicidal ideation and/or severe agitation is common.

Ehrlichia/Anaplasma are bacteria that are related that come in both acute and chronic forms. Acutely, symptoms occur abruptly and cause a high fever, muscle pain, headaches, elevated liver enzymes, and occasionally a low white blood cell (WBC) count. The chronic form causes headaches and muscle soreness, knife-like pains, persistent low WBC, and unexplained elevated liver enzymes. Ehrlichia can cause pain in the hips and shoulders.

Mycoplasma Fermentans is a bacteria which causes Gulf War syndrome, exacerbates the underlying symptom complex a person is experiencing, and is probably responsible for part of chronic relapse. Unrelenting fatigue and subtle neurological dysfunction are part of the picture. When the sickest and most chronic Lyme patients are separated from the rest, Mycoplasma is usually present. It causes signs of autoimmunity or symptoms of autoimmune diseases. It interferes with metabolism, causes cell damage, and competes for nutrients.

Rocky Mountain Spotted Fever is a ricketsial infection that has an abrupt onset. A spotted, large rash is common and is found on the hands and feet, as well as other parts of the body. Headache, fever, and body pains are typical. A low WBC count and elevated liver enzymes occur. This infection can be fatal.

Other bacteria to consider are Typhus, Chlamydia pneumonia (not the sexually transmitted disease), and Tularemia. Q-Fever and Tick paralysis are rickettsia and can be found as co-infections.

Parasites include Babesia, already discussed, and other piroplasms, filiariasis, amoebas, and giardia. Many of these are found in the intestinal tract and can have a profound effect on the immune system and quality of life. Intestinal parasites can cause severe fatigue, weight loss, and abdominal symptoms that are often diagnosed as Irritable Bowel Syndrome. When you see the word "syndrome," it is a clue that what is causing the symptom complex is unknown, but the complex is seen with regularity.

Viruses are numerous. They are most often opportunistic infections that flare up when the immune system is compromised, as with CLD. They include many different Herpes viruses (HHV- 1, 2, 6, 8,), Cytomegalo (CMV) Virus, Epstein Bar Virus (EBV), St Louis Encephalopathies, West Nile Virus, XMRV Virus, and other viral encephaolpathies.

Fungal infections, like Candida and other fungi, can invade the intestinal tract, especially with long-term antibiotic therapy. Symptoms can be similar to parasite infections.

Many factors need to be assessed when diagnosing CLD. They include:

A. Inflammation.

B. Immune dysfunction.

C. Toxicity—especially multiple chemical sensitivity, environmental illness, heavy metals, mold, and neurotoxins.

D. Allergies.

E. Nutritional and enzyme deficiencies.

F. Cellular dysfunction.

G. Psychological Stress: Abuse, Post-Traumatic Stress Disorder, rape, depression, anxiety, Obsessive Compulsive Disorder.

H. Endocrine dysfunction: including thyroid, adrenal, pituitary, and sex hormone deficiency, as well as Vitamin D deficiency.

I. Sleep Disorders.

J.   Gastrointestinal issues, like Leaky Gut, Dysbiosis, Candida, Colitis, and cancer.

K.   Drug Addiction/Use.

As you can see, there are many considerations when diagnosing chronic illness, especially CLD. Many of these issues play into the complexity of treating someone who has been infected, usually, for several years before they find a Lyme-literate practitioner. The infections have had years to establish themselves in the various tissues of the body, and it is necessary to pull them out to effect a cure. It can take years.

SYMPTOM CHECK LIST: Lyme Disease Evaluation

General
Fever
Night Sweats
Fatigue, lack of endurance
Unexplained weight gain/loss
Generalized, unprovoked pain
Migratory pain

Head, Face, Neck
Headache, mild or severe
Facial flushing
Pressure in head
Jaw pain or stiffness
Unexplained hair loss
Dental problems/pain (unexplained)
Twitching of facial muscles

Stiff or painful neck
Facial paralysis (Bell's Palsy)
Sore throat, hoarseness
Tingling of nose, tongue, cheek

Eyes/Vision and Ears/Hearing
Double or blurry vision
Difficulty with night vision
Increased floating spots
Pain in eyes or swelling around eyes
Oversensitivity to light
Flashing lights/peripheral waves/ phantom images
Change in color vision
Decreased hearing in one or both ears
Pain in ears, over sensitivity to sounds
Auditory hallucinations

Gastrointestinal and Genito-urinary Systems
Upset stomach (nausea/pain)/ heartburn
Recurrent vomiting
Diarrhea/ constipation
Irritable bladder or interstitial cystitis
Testicular or pelvic pain
Decreased libido
Unexplained menstrual irregularity
Symptoms worse with menses? Yes No
Unexplained milk production

Musculoskeletal System
Bone pain, joint pain or swelling
Carpal Tunnel syndrome
Stiffness of joints, back, neck
Frequent tendonitis, tennis elbow
Muscle pain or cramps, muscle spasms
Sore soles, especially in the morning

Respiratory and Circulatory Systems
Shortness of breath, cough
Endocarditis, myocarditis, heart failure
Chest pain or rib soreness
Peripheral vascular abnormalities
Rhythm disturbances—extra beats
 Heart block, palpitations

Psychological
Mood swings, irritability
Feeling as if you are losing your mind
Over-emotional reactions, crying easily
Depression
Bi-polar disorder
Panic attacks, anxiety
Obsessive compulsive disorder
Psychosis

Mental Capability
Memory loss (short or long term)
Going to the wrong place

Disorientation (getting or feeling lost)
Confusion, difficulty thinking
Forgetting how-to perform simple tasks
Difficulty with concentration or reading
Dementia

Nervous System
Burning, stabbing, aching or shock sensations
Lightheadedness, fainting
Numbness, tingling, pinpricks
Increased motion sickness
Peripheral neuropathies
Abnormalities of vision, hearing, smell, taste, or touch
Muscle weakness
Muscle atrophy or partial paralysis
Muscle twitching
Speech difficulty (slurred or slow)
Stammering speech
Word searching, misspeaking
Poor balance
Dizziness
Difficulty walking, gait problems
Tremors
Seizures
Sleep problems: excessive sleep, insomnia. Sleep apnea, narcolepsy, unusual sleeping behaviors

Decreased alcohol tolerance?   Yes   No

With the variety of symptoms that are caused by CLD, it is easy to see why a provider who is unfamiliar and uneducated about these infections would believe that someone was crazy and making up their problems. To a Lyme-literate provider, these symptoms tell a story and lead to a diagnosis.

4: MORE STORIES

THIS STORY IS TOLD BY Mona in her own words. I leave it untouched as it gives you, the reader, an inkling of the complexity of CLD, and how this affects someone with these infections. Mona is amazing and full of light and positive energy, despite her illness.

MONA'S STORY - HOW I CAME INTO THE LYMELIGHT

"Four years ago, I was a successful civil rights lawyer with a passion for life, the outdoors, and explosive energy. Now, I'm attached to an IV pole, in my PJ's, and on a couch. I need my parents, friends, and others for care. Why? I have late-stage Lyme disease or CLD. I have gone through 25 months of often excruciating treatment, which has taken away my independence, ability to function, my career, my ability to enjoy all the sports I love, and a full social life. But I am still ready to keep fighting.

How did I get Lyme? Where did I get it? What were my symptoms? How was I diagnosed?

My story is long and complex, but like most late-stage Lyme cases, it involves a great deal of misunderstanding on the part of the mainstream medical community, over $100,000 in credit card debt to pay for my medical bills, dozens of doctors, hospital visits, and tests, more emotional and physical suffering than I ever thought I could handle, family drama, loss of years of my life, and a ton of ups and downs.

I hope I can help even ONE person who reads this who is sick with Lyme (but doesn't know it and, sadly, there is a high probability they don't know it—the average number of doctors Lyme patients see before getting an accurate diagnosis is TEN, and at this point, the disease is drilled deep into your body), experiencing "ambiguous" symptoms that mainstream doctors cannot diagnose, that I can save from experiencing losing years of their life. If someone had educated me earlier, or if any of the 14 doctors I saw over 2 years at top institutions like UCSF and other major hospitals had properly diagnosed me, I would have been able to treat this disease with a much better fighting chance. The longer Lyme goes undiagnosed, the farther it goes into all systems of your body, the more intolerable the symptoms become, and the longer, harder, and more expensive treatment is. And the more difficult remission is.

The worst part of this disease is that your symptoms and level of ability to function can literally change by the day, the hour, even by the minute. Up, down, up, down... I was on different treatments, addressing different co-infections, and when you ignore one, another creeps up. Then you need to knock that one down. Then Lyme creeps back in. You have to keep changing the game, the drugs you use because the bacteria get smart, and figure out what works. Then the treatment itself, like chemotherapy, makes you sicker than sick. Then you feel a day or two or even a week or month of improvement. Hallelujah!! Boom, then you're bed ridden for 3 days. It makes NO sense, it is not linear, and one just has to accept this as long as you know you're generally trending upwards.

I love my parents, but even after watching me battle this disease and learning all about it, they still ask me, "What happened? You were fine just 3 hours ago!" What happened? It's called Lyme. NO RHYME OR REASON.

One minute you're standing up in Target (after browsing around for only 15 minutes), and 3 minutes later you are scooting on your ASS down the aisle at Target while people stare at you because you can no longer walk or stand up without collapsing from weakness, and they think I look totally healthy (yes, this happened to me and I had to scoot to the front and page my mom in the store to come get me, it was like being 5 years old again). Then you're crying in the car and have traumatic memories of Target. But I digress.

The rollercoaster of this disease is SO frustrating because you NEVER know what your body is going to do on any given day. For my psyche, it is torture. My body and soul get pulled and tugged up and down constantly, and all I know is that the IMMENSE uncertainty (will I be able to walk outside today? go to dinner with a friend? make a meal? read? or flat line in bed with sunglasses on under the covers, hoping I will die in my sleep?) throws my heart into a fearful melting; my spirit may be lifted briefly and then washed away by a terrible tidal wave for days, weeks, or months. Then I will feel better for weeks and amazed at how much progress I've made so quickly.

WHEN I WAS DIAGNOSED

I was diagnosed with Lyme disease (which is more properly called Lyme Borreliosis Complex nowadays, because it is really so many other things than just Lyme) in July of 2008. I was ecstatic when I got the test results in the mail.

The test was ordered by Dr. Heyman, a brilliant University of Michigan doctor professor who worked with the famous holistic Dr. Andrew Weil and was an expert in chronic diseases. He spent, at our first appointment, 4 HOURS with my mom and his pharmacologist, going through my three binders of labs/medical records that I brought, sitting with me explaining all the potential causes of my "mystery illness." He sent my blood to Igenex. Most Lyme patients get their blood tested for Lyme via Igenex or another famous lab out East. Igenex is the gold standard, from what I understand.

I had been sick on and off for over 2 years prior to that and disabled to the point I had to stop working 8 months earlier. Finally, AN ANSWER!!! Lyme. Yes, a plan!! No more mystery. Treat the Lyme, and move on with life!! Woohoo, I thought. I had been to over 14 doctors in 2 years—specialists all over the country— lucky that my parents would fund my decision to seek out holistic, integrative, and traditional doctors to find an answer to what had been plaguing me since late 2005. I remember driving to the Rose Garden in Golden Gate Park just a few minutes from my place, and calling my best friend, Emily, and told her the news. I was excited to enter this new chapter and end it quickly. I was anxious, but hopeful.

Little did I know the treatment of this disease was THE most difficult, painful, and long thing I would ever do in my life.

WHEN I STARTED GOING DOWNHILL

Below I jump back in time to 2005 when the earliest symptoms started appearing, but I had NO idea they were connected to Lyme until later.

It was 2007 that REALLY took me down. Spring of 2007, I wasn't feeling OK. But I could still manage to function for the most part. Struggled through it, but I did it. Dizziness, vertigo spells coming and going, and weakness. I was often lightheaded and tired after exercise and hikes. I had horrible migraines that lasted weeks and really bad menstrual cycles, along with fatigue that was getting worse.

*Quick note: for those of you who don't know me, before I fell ill, I was a hyper ball of energy, passionate about everything, smiling, dancing, snowboarding, rock climbing, hiking, climbing mountains, travelling, surfing, volunteering, I was a Type A work hard, play hard, love life person. I co-founded a non-profit (www.sparksf.org) in 2004, finished law school, passed the California Bar Exam. I was not sitting on the side-line of life. Then, I got side-lined, and oh did my perspective of life change. I haven't exercised in exactly THREE years.

Summer 2007: I start a new job, dream job at a non-profit law foundation, litigating fair housing and predatory lending in Silicon Valley. My commute is 3 hours round-trip, and I work long hours, and am under a GREAT deal of stress. I LOVE the job, but I was overwhelmed, huge caseload. Took on so many cases, delved into a whole new area of law, learning about state and federal litigation rules, depositions, trial, settlement conferences, arbitration, plus federal banking laws, state and federal housing laws, was saturated with so much new information that I was having nightmares about it many nights. The first week, I could barely make it to work all 5 days. I couldn't get out of bed the first Friday and had to call in sick. I couldn't WALK to my bathroom without using EVERY ounce of energy in my body. I knew something was wrong.

Tons of visits to numerous endocrinologists and chronic fatigue specialists and naturopaths and homeopaths ensued. I find out I have some endocrine problems, hypothyroidism (which can make you really ill and extremely fatigued), adrenal fatigue, and all kinds of imbalances in my hormones that were making me lose weight really fast, sleep 16 hours a night on weekends, barely able to do anything on those weekend days, trudging through work, a complete insomniac, heart palpitations, chest pain, an emotional wreck (I remember getting a ticket on Cal-train on the way to work one day and getting off the train and hysterically crying like a baby), and, most detrimental to my career, totally unable to work my brain.

It was like a huge fog swallowed my brain slowly, and pretty soon I was at work all cracked out on meds the doctors had tried me out on (some various unpleasant protocols for vertiginous migraines), until I was spending afternoons under my desk having to lay down and my colleague was asking if she needed to drive me home.

Then came the kicker—I thought one of our MANY cases had settled. I was sure of it. I remember reading an email from our assistant counsel. At our weekly meetings to review the status of all cases, I mentioned this case had settled. They, in fact, had not. Nobody had settled. I don't know if I was running on 3 hours of sleep or had completely lost my short-term memory, but I knew I had to take medical leave and figure out what REALLY was going on with my health. My boss, an AMAZING woman with a heart of gold and extreme passion for helping the underserved, took over for me on many projects, despite the fact that her workload was already saturated. Sadly, she was in fact getting sick with a "mystery illness" at the same time, as well.

I spoke with her and we agreed it would be best to take medical leave, rest, go through all the doctors I needed to figure out what was wrong. I said I'd be back in 1 month, no problem. She said take 3 months, do what you need to get healthy, and then come back. I never went back. They held my job for 6 months, but by that time, I was sicker than I was before and still had no REAL answers. I was DEVASTATED. My good friend and ex-boyfriend, Fred, had helped me realize that I had to quit, I had to give up the first of many things I would be giving up. Giving up my dream job was crushing to me and my sense of where I belonged in the world. Only 2 years out of law school, 31, and already disabled? I cried for days but knew it was the right thing to do. I felt my goals and dreams of practicing civil rights and human rights law and helping those with no voice swirl down the drain.

In this time, sadly, my boss, found out her mystery illness was pancreatic cancer and she quickly underwent treatment. This amazingly generous, giving, and intelligent woman, who I never saw again after our conversation in November 2007, in her 30's, with two little kids and an adoring husband, passed away in the spring of 2008 from pancreatic cancer.

After I quit my job, new symptoms began to appear in 2008, for example, a 6-week bout of excruciating joint pain and fevers. I'd never experienced anything like it in my life. I could barely move my wrists, or open a door knob or even cut some butter. I was staying with my parents in Michigan, and my mom held me while I just cried hysterically waiting for the pain to pass. It was like someone was sledgehammering my joints. That passed, but my fatigue and other symptoms were still lurking heavily.

FLASHBACK

Flashback to late 2005:Finished and passed the CA Bar exam in the summer, flew to South America to travel with a good friend to celebrate, was outside in the mountains of Peru and Ecuador and ended up with over 80 bites on my legs that took weeks to subside. I never thought anything of it. Personally, still think I got bit in Northern CA. When I returned to the US, I had a hard break-up with a boyfriend.

Started working as an attorney, but experienced strange nightly panic/terror attacks out of nowhere. Had NO idea where these were coming from, but I woke up hyperventilating many times, almost to the point I would pass out. Fingers and arms would get tingly and numb. Thought it was related to stress, or break-up, it passed after a few months. (You will see why this is Lyme-related later).

2006 UP AND DOWN

I felt okay after the panic attacks passed, but I did get these weird transient vertigo migraine things that lasted days occasionally, coming and going and scaring the shit out of me. My neurologists always attested them to residual migraines from the dissected vertebral artery (head trauma) I endured from a chiropractor in 2002 (which nearly paralyzed me, more on that below). They didn't come too often. I was doing great in February 2006, I remember going to Tahoe with my sister, brother-in-law, niece, and snowboarded hard all day, drinking at night with the crew of friends up there. A few weeks later, I had to take an antibiotic - Flagyl - for stomach issues. It was a 10 day-course, but the day after I stopped the meds, I IMMEDIATELY went into a horrendous downward spiral where I woke up and LITERALLY felt like I was falling to the ground and being pulled down to the left.

Any time I moved, the world spun in circles, went up, down, I felt like throwing up, felt like my head wasn't screwed on, a horrible sense of disassociation from my body, dizziness, vertigo, confusion, anxiety, nausea. The only thing I could liken it to was the symptoms after I had the dissected artery in 2002 and ended up in the ICU for 7 days. I was fatigued and couldn't even move from my bed. When my eyes moved, the world went up and down. There was no way to describe what I was feeling other than it felt like I had overdosed on some horrible hallucinogenic drug. My friend, Nicole, was visiting from out of town and I felt so horrible that during her visit, I couldn't get out of bed. She came to the ER with me on her short visit to SF. That would be the first of MANY visits to the ER with many friends.

What was happening to me? I could barely stand up straight that day; it was so odd and SO scary. I could only hypothesize that it had something to do with my old dissected vertebral artery injury. At the ER, I told them I was worried about the artery and could it have re-dissected? Since so little is known about follow up of dissected vertebral arteries (one of my neurologists told me I was "famous" for having that injury as it was so rare...gee thanks), it was unclear to the ER docs if I had re-dissected the artery. But since I hadn't done anything lately (yoga poses, car accidents, tumbles down the mountain) that would have likely reinjured my head, the chance was unlikely. They didn't want to subject me to more CT scans of my brain since I'd already had way more than necessary for my age. They said to follow up with a neurologist, but that there was no immediate danger.

Great, on the one hand. But this thing, this monster of weirdness that came out of NOWHERE, put me out of work and in bed for 3 weeks, and took over 6 MONTHS to subside. Still wasn't diagnosed with Lyme, just living in some weird limbo of illness. I lost 15 lbs., could barely eat, and was nauseated and exhausted. I went to every doctor, got tested for every possible scenario, and was then told by the top migraine specialist/neurologist at UCSF that I was experiencing rare vertiginous migraines, most likely as a residual from the artery incident. OK, I thought. So they thought putting me on some migraine medications, including Diamox (a medication for high altitude), would do something to alleviate the imbalances and problems in my head. *NOPE, they made me sicker.* I was so ill on those meds, the side effects and the combination of strange medications made my sensitive and weak little body even sicker.

I finally went to an amazing naturopathic and homeopathic doctor who found out via testing I had heavy metal toxicity and some other issues that she addressed with holistic treatments, homeopathy, and nutritional supplementation. I got better about 6 months later, to the point I could function, work, and exercise. But I was never really back to normal.

FATE STEPPED IN

Mid-2008: My mom was flying back from San Francisco (where I live) to Michigan and randomly struck a conversation with a woman next to her on the plane. My mother makes conversation with almost everyone she meets; she is a microbiologist, an entrepreneur, business woman, and social butterfly at her core. During this time (early 2008), I had been diagnosed, by one of the top chronic fatigue syndrome (CFS)/hormone balance centers in Los Angeles, with CFS/fibromyalgia and adrenal fatigue (which is another condition that mainstream doctors don't recognize or know how to treat).

Anyhow, as fate would have it (and there is no doubt universal forces were at work here), the woman's daughter-in-law was so ill for over a year that she had to quit working, could barely function as a human being and had seen an amazing integrative doctor, Dr. Andrew Heyman in Ann Arbor, Michigan, who worked with the famous Dr. Andrew Weil and who also had a medical degree and professorship at the University of Michigan. I didn't see Dr. Heyman right away, but went to him a few months later, when I kept getting worse and had to go stay with my parents. He was my angel; he diagnosed my Lyme and brought my illness a NAME!

LYME TREATMENT: BEGIN!! August 2008

After the brilliant and compassionate Dr. Heyman diagnosed me with Lyme FINALLY in the summer of 2008, he told me I had to see an infectious disease Lyme specialist in SF, where I was living. Dr. Heyman, in private practice and faculty at the University of Michigan Medical School, sat with me for almost FOUR HOURS at my first appointment (can you find ANY doctor who will do that nowadays?), parsed through my hundreds of medical records and labs and symptoms with his pharmacologist. They ran a number of other tests and posited theories. Their Lyme theory was correct. He confirmed what I heard already through the Lyme patient grapevine—that there were only 2 labs in the country that had accurate lab testing for Lyme Disease, one of them being the famous Igenex Labs in Palo Alto (where almost every Lyme patient in CA gets their Lyme labs done; other labs are useless). After my labs came back blaringly positive from Igenex in July 2008, I was ecstatic and ready to tackle head on this "thing" that consumed my life for almost three years and now had a NAME. LYME!!!!!!!!!

SWELL TO THE BEGINNINGS OF HELL

I got in with Dr. S, in San Francisco, one of the most famous Lyme specialists in the world, who had treated numerous celebrities, including Amy Tan, author of the *Joy Luck Club* (www.canlyme.com/amy). I didn't know anything about Lyme; Dr. S told me we would START by treating the co-infection Babesia. Later on, we'd get to other co-infections and the Lyme. He explained what herxing was, which I'd already read about online. I took my meds, went home, and waited for the fun to start. The first few weeks were rough but not terrible, and then I was slammed. The more Babesia and Lyme I killed, the more I herxed and the sicker I became.

I went back to Michigan for a few months to stay with my parents, and was so incredibly ill I had to CRAWL, literally, to get to the bathroom 5 feet away. My mom would feed me while I lay on the ground. I didn't get OUT of my pyjamas OR leave the house once in 3 weeks. I was more exhausted than I ever imagined possible. It felt like a 400-lb. gorilla was literally crushing me and I had to push him off with my little strength to move. I had vertigo, migraines, and crazy neurological symptoms (remember a herx is often an exacerbation of the symptoms to very scary degrees as the bugs die off and release toxic cytokines that are trying to leave your body) where I would just lay in bed with my hand on my head and see crazy visual blurs bombarding my head.

I lay in my pyjamas at the top of the stairs and my mom would spoon feed me and put water in my throat. It was AWFUL. Awful doesn't even begin to describe the surreal hell I lived in at that time.

Again, I thought Lyme was no big deal like most of society, just a disease that you treat with some antibiotics for a few months and then on your way. I was so wrong on so many levels. In my worst nightmare, I never would have imagined that the treatment and the process of eradicating this disease was worse than the disease, so much so that I would call it "a gruelling triathlon that lasted years" an understatement; it was more like a chemotherapy of mind, body, spirit, and existence that lasts years and goes up and down a few thousand times, sometimes within a day, or a week, or months, a waterboarding of every piece of your soul, a shredding of your body, an annihilation of your cognitive abilities, a torture chamber of the loneliest and scariest places you have ever visited in your mind. Nobody holding your hand, nobody knowing what to tell you, just lying in a hospital bed or bed at home wondering if you are in fact dying, and if you're not dying, could God or the Universe or someone up there just kill you now. A hell I would NEVER imagined possible.

I've endured a lot of physical pain. I've been an athlete all my life, enduring back injuries, falls, car accidents, concussions, and even breaking my pelvis in a snowboarding competition in 2002. Later that fall, my first year of law school, I saw a chiropractor one evening, passed out in his office, ended up in the ER and found out he had dissected my vertebral artery—torn the artery in the back of my neck connected to my brain. I was lucky I didn't have a stroke, get paralyzed, or die from that incident. I was rushed to the ICU and on blood thinners and heavy narcotics for a year. The physical pain is hard to deal with, but when you have your mind, you can get through that. But add to that physical pain the inability to often have a clear mind, and the game of surviving this disease becomes akin to climbing Mt. Everest.

Whenever anyone asks me about my symptoms, I get too irritated to list them all and go through this enormously convoluted and complex story. Sometimes I describe it like trying to climb Mt. Everest, getting close, sliding down in some painful fashion, and trying to climb it over and over and over. And over. And over. And over and over and over again. And you're still not there.

Back to being at home in Michigan...I couldn't sleep, I just lay there being tortured by monsters in my brain from the die-off (herx) from the treatment. Once I told my doctor that it felt like my head had to vomit all the time; he said that was a great description of what his Lyme patients felt. Then came the depression. Oh boy nobody told me about this. I had joined the Lyme support group online and went to an in-person meeting once in San Francisco, but I had NO idea that complete mental breakdowns where you throw yourself on the kitchen floor crying for HOURS EVERY night for months were part of the herx. Dr. S never told me!! I called his office because it was so bad I felt like I was losing it and he never called back. That was unacceptable. So I changed docs.

Bottom line: I was herxing WAY too hard. I didn't know though. From the millions of Lyme support group posts I read online and research I had done, I understood that the name of the game was herxing, which meant torture. Think chemotherapy of sorts - pain means gain. But then even Dr. S told me this was too much herxing, which basically means the drugs are killing off the disease at SUCH a high rate that my body couldn't keep up with getting rid of it (this is why 8 million detox supplements and routines are essential).

Then you're just recycling dead bugs (Lyme and co-infections) in your blood and getting sicker. It is dangerous.

*Side note on adrenal fatigue for those interested: Chronic fatigue syndrome (CFS)/fibromyalgia are, IMO, umbrella terms to being very ill and not knowing why. A host of reasons can cause CFS, and adrenal fatigue was one of my causes. Adrenal fatigue was devastating to my immune system - I slept 16 hours a night and could barely stay awake 7 hours a day or exercise without feeling like collapsing. My emotional state was a mess and I could remember NOTHING, precipitating the need for me to take medical leave from my highly coveted job as a civil rights attorney. Adrenal fatigue, FYI, is an imbalance, brought on by stress most often, toxicity, environmental pollutants, and other factors, that prevents your body's ability to make cortisol. Cortisol is what you need to literally get out of bed in the morning. Cortisol is what is released during the human "fight or flight" phenomenon. Adrenal fatigue is a complex condition with tons of books written on it. Dr. Wilson's Adrenal Fatigue Site is one example. The most common symptoms of adrenal fatigue are: unrelenting fatigue, horrible response to stress, exercise intolerance, depression, anxiety, insomnia, poor memory and concentration, low blood sugar, dizziness and low blood pressure.

NEXT ROUTE: MEDICINAL HERBS WITH LYME NATUROPATH

After experiencing 3 months of literal torture on every level in every cell of my body, I saw Dr. A up in Santa Rosa in October 2008, who had been HIGHLY recommended as the best Lyme doctor who would combine holistic and traditional (drugs) treatment. I saw him, and he wanted to take me off the meds and let my body play catch up. He told me I was too sick from the herxing, and needed to let that toxic sludge get out of my body, and put me on herbs for a while, and then return to drugs again when the time was right. Although I am VERY holistic in my approach to medicine, and actually am not a huge fan of Western medicine's pill pushing regime, I was still apprehensive about these herbs. Herbs? That will kill these infections?

I took the leap of faith. His office was PACKED with very ill Lyme patients from all over the state, and he was compassionate and LISTENED. He also put me on a number of adjunct holistic protocols to heal my gut, work on my methylation pathways (a genetic defect in detoxification process that most Lyme patients have), address any parasites, heavy metals, or other toxic elements that invade Lyme patients so easily because our immune systems have been totally whacked down by the Lyme. That is HOW powerful this disease is. Herbs that you could slowly work up in doses. I herxed on the herbs. A LOT!! Holy shit, who knew? They were working; I did this for about 6 months. I started feeling better! Then the Lyme started creeping in, and the herbs were not powerful enough. I needed the big guns: drugs and then IV drugs and my body knew it.

Dr. A put me back on oral antibiotic treatment for Bartonella, and I made some progress in the summer of 2009. Back and forth between Michigan and San Francisco I went. I returned to SF in July of 2009 right after my 32nd birthday. The treatment I was on became unbearable. I was in so much pain my friend carried me up the stairs and stuck a Vicodin in my mouth and my oxygen tank in my nostrils. My Babesia was back (I could tell because its tell-tale symptom was air hunger, literally feeling like you are choking and cannot breathe). On my flight to SF, I thought I was going to die. Plane trips are notoriously hard on Lyme patients because the hypoxic environment. Babesia makes it feel like you cannot breathe.

Got back on Babesia treatment (Western drugs) and within a week I was OFF my oxygen tank and felt amazing. As I said, it's a balancing act with the co-infections and Lyme.

NEW LIFE!

Switched to Dr. G in July 2009, partner of Dr. S, and she put me on Babesia and other protocol, and I felt great for a few months. I was driving around, getting groceries, going on dates, even went to a bar once and sang on stage! Who WAS this girl? I hadn't seen her in years. It was amazing to feel parts of my old self re-emerge. One day I walked 50 minutes, which is HUGE for me. HUGE!!! I was having dinner with friends, still taking my naps and needing a ton of rest, but really functioning at a level I had not in over 2 ½ years. Was ecstatic, and then went to Michigan...

Stayed there for about 11 months...saw Dr. J out east, got my PICC line put in my arm/heart on March 1, 2010. 2010 was very rough. VERY rough. IV is not easy and very intense. I'm back in San Francisco now, as of September 10, 2010!"

Presently Mona has stopped treatment with IV medications. She remains hopeful that she will get well. A combination of pharmaceutical and nutritional supplements has improved her quality of life and helped her handle the treatment. But the ups and downs remain. Her positive attitude and strong spirit carry her through the rough spots.

Below is an article written by one of my clients with Chronic Lyme Disease (CLD). I include it here to exemplify some of the struggle. Her words say it so well:

"The recent ad by Vector control is commendable. Awareness of the dangers of tick bites in our beautiful region is something we need to focus on as a community. How many of us know that when we hike and camp in Northern California, there are virtual "dirty needles" littering our parks? These "dirty needles" are ticks, and they aren't just lying around waiting for "the unsuspecting" to accidentally trip over them; they are literally stalking us humans (and deer and any other blood carrying creature they can spot). They are

traveling out to the tips of plants and leaves with their arms outstretched, waiting to grab onto the next being that brushes past. This offensive move is called "questing." Once attached, it is true, as the Vector control ad points out, a person can possibly become inoculated by this "dirty needle" with the pernicious and genetically complex bug, Borrelia burgdorferi, known as "Lyme."

But do dirty needles only carry one pathogen? Very good, class! No they do not! Ticks have been inoculating themselves into mice, rats, birds, raccoons, deer and every other hapless creature which may be out hiking in the park. This means that a tick bite most likely carries several pathogenic organisms, from viruses to worms to protozoans. This is why there is a move to rename what has been called "Lyme" disease to a more comprehensive designation that includes a constellation of infections.

As the Vector Control ad points out, taking yourself to the physician with symptoms of fatigue, malaise, joint pain, unexplained neurological and cardiac irregularities may well be an appropriate course of action. Unfortunately, when Lyme is the concern, calling up the local physician is sometimes like dialing up for Batman and getting Joker. As pervasive as Lyme disease is in our county, there are precious few Lyme specialists, none of whom take insurance, who will seriously treat or properly refer someone experiencing Lyme.

The sufferer is told that there are two paradigms and that most MDs do not ascribe to the "chronic Lyme" paradigm. Can you imagine having a breast removed for cancer and then returning with a lump on the other breast and being told that since you were already treated for breast cancer, you no longer have it? The reality is *that current diagnostic and antibiotic protocols are inadequate, and are an insufficient match for not only the Lyme bug, which is infinitely more genetically complex than syphilis, but also for the multiple co-infections that do not respond to the standard antibiotic protocol. For example, a malaria-like protozoan called Babesia is commonly present as a co-infection. This pathogen on its own can actually kill the vulnerable, children, the elderly and the immune compromised. Babesia, like malaria, requires its own unique classes of antibiotics and antimalarials. It should be suspected in every case of Lyme.*

Lyme sufferers are routinely being ignored, misdiagnosed and refused by their physicians. Their disease conditions are going unchecked, causing many to suffer irreparable neurological and joint damage. In fact, any system in the body, including hormonal, thyroid and cardiac, is prey to a Lyme infection.

It would be unthinkable to ignore a malignancy in any system of the body. When cancer is suspected, the proper specialist is engaged. That specialist is part of the medical system and has devoted many hours to mastering the nuances of cancer. Most infectious disease doctors are no match for the complexities of Lyme and associated co-infections. The Infectious Disease Society guidelines are inadequate for both diagnosis and treatment. This is because both diagnosis and treatment of Lyme are better managed by monitoring the clinical picture, rather than a dogmatic reliance on testing which has proven to render false negatives. In fact, the revered "bull's-eye-rash" is now thought to occur only when one is reinfected, whence the body produces a pronounced immune response in the form of an expanding rash. Only 30 % of positive Lyme cases can sport such a rash, so fixating on presence of a rash is just plain ludicrous.

It is time for courage. Anyone who brings up the word "Lyme" in a social group or place of business will more often than not cull horror stories of this friend or that relative, tucked away in bed for the last eight years, unable to move due to pain, or worse, unable to think clearly. Why courage? It is time to render these ones who have been cast out by the medical community the proper care that anyone with cancer is afforded. A Lyme sufferer deserves a proper referral to a Lyme specialist, who is covered under their medical insurance plan, just as a cancer patient would receive such a referral to a cancer specialist.

Lyme disease and associated co-infection management is a specialty all its own. Lyme requires complex management of many issues: multiple co-infections; multiple affected body systems, including hormonal manifestations; management of overload of cytokines which on their own can cause organ damage through increasing inflammation; and yes, Virginia, management of toxin release in presence of profound "die off," just as in any other pathogenic disease which can cause damaging neurotoxic release. Let's take courage as a medical community and also as a broader community of folks who have "most of us" heard of someone struggling with Lyme. Lyme patients deserve to have appropriate and accessible specialized care, as much as any other person suffering with unique disease.

Thank you, Vector Control, for bringing Lyme "out of the closet" once again!" -Gretchen Daniels, RN, BSN Santa Rosa"

Gretchen has worked in the Western Health Care system for over 30 years. When she contracted Lyme disease, she tried repeatedly to get help from the system she trusted. It was a shock and extremely distressing to her that she was belittled and ignored until her disease had progressed to a point where it became chronic and more challenging to treat. It took her more than a year to start treatment, which put her into the chronic category of Lyme.

AMANDA'S STORY

Nothing is worse than watching your child suffer day after day.

Amanda, my daughter, is 36 years old. She was two years old when we found a tick on the back of her neck. Then at 15 years old, Amanda got bitten on her breast. There was a rash, the classic bull's eye, and a black area surrounding the bite. I know now that this means multiple co-infections, but then I was a nurse working in homecare and hospice and knew nothing about TBD—neither did the physicians who saw the bite reaction. Symptoms were subtle for several years. Frequent respiratory infections, including pneumonia, aches and pains, gastrointestinal symptoms of diarrhea and vomiting occurred often. She was easily carsick and had a hard time sitting in the back of a car. Then about seven years ago, Amanda had an unexplained blood clot in her lung. She was in the hospital for several days. Test after test showed nothing. Finally, the respiratory specialist discovered an obscure genetic clotting disorder and placed her on a blood thinner.

This turned out to be a good move as more clots would have followed without the medication.

Amanda has always had emotional issues. She was raped and molested as a preteen, and we always thought her emotional problems were related to Post Traumatic Stress Disorder. Panic and anxiety attacks started about 10 years ago and have gotten progressively worse.

Then 1-½ years ago, Amanda contracted pneumonia again, then H1N1 virus, and the last straw was exposure to black mold, which was later found in the ceiling above her bed. She became bedridden. She couldn't breathe or eat. It was then that the diagnosis of CLD was made. Now, over 20 years infected, she is severely sensitive to any treatment due to the effect of the die-off and the toxins produced by the bacteria and the hyper-reactivity of her immune system. The treatment pushes her to the point of vomiting, and she can't stop. Her pain goes beyond a 10/10. She becomes dehydrated, and off to the ER we go.

For the past nine months, Amanda has been in the ER 14 times and hospitalized five times. We have tried several different ER's, and they are all the same. How she is treated depends on the physician on call. Four times, the MD inadequately treated her dehydration and failed to give her enough medicine to stop her vomiting and control her pain. They do not believe her diagnosis of CLD and think it doesn't exist. One said giving her Dilaudid, a potent narcotic, would only make her euphoric, so he refused to give it. Instead, he gave her a potent anti-inflammatory which causes GI bleeding. He limited her IV fluid to 1 ½ liters, when she needed at least 5 to 6 liters to be able to urinate again, and sent her home, still vomiting. We were back the next day. It took 6 liters of fluid and multiple doses of medicine to control her symptoms, and she was admitted to the hospital.

After two days in the hospital, another physician sent her home before she was taking oral fluids. We were back in the ER two days later, and that time, she spent 5 days in the hospital. Doctor after doctor refused to believe she had CLD, instead calling in a psychologist and recommending therapy. It had to be all in her head.

About two months ago, Amanda and I visited a man who is enlightened, completely without ego. Robert spent an hour with Amanda, helping to facilitate a healing response. When Amanda walked into the room, she was leaning on me and could barely stand. He had her close her eyes and lean her head back, gently talking with her. Robert told her that she was going to give him all her pain and nausea. He said that he would take the pain, but not keep it, rather "giving it to the trees because they love shit!" For almost the entire hour, Robert went to every place in Amanda's body that hurt, which was extensive. At the end, she came out of the meditative state she was in and remarked that she felt no pain or nausea. When we left, Amanda was able to walk gracefully and with energy out of the house. About two hours later, she felt a deep exhaustion and went to sleep, and slept for over eight hours. Upon awakening, she began to purge all the debris that had moved from the inside of her cells, and this caused her to begin vomiting. It was too much detoxifying too quickly for such a sensitive body. We ended up in the hospital, and she spent five days there.

However, after a few weeks, Amanda's energy improved and she felt hunger again. Her need for narcotics was reduced by half, and her nausea had improved. These are miraculous changes.

Sitting in the ER this last time, in the hallway, was, once again, a distressing experience. The MD was someone we had dealt with once before while Amanda was hospitalized. He had told Amanda that I was impeding her care. Then, this time in the ER, he asked me to leave. The arrogance of young physicians is astounding. I was told by a hospital medical director that young doctors have to be right. What a joke! In health care, we learn that 90% of the diagnosis is gleaned from the clinical history given by the patient and their family. Who better to give the history? Add to that my professional expertise, and it becomes stupid to choose to disregard this avenue of information. Amanda was belittled and received only 2 liters of fluid, rather than the necessary 6 liters. She was denied needed medicines to bring her symptoms under control at this doctor's whim. Finally, she was discharged before she had stopped vomiting and was left in a wheelchair sitting in the waiting room to be retrieved. She couldn't hold her head up, she was so weak. Once back at our house, she continued to vomit. This experience exemplifies what many with these infections endure when they are forced to interact in the Western Health Care System.

I sent a letter to the medical director of the hospital and included numerous references on articles in respected medical journals on the persistence of these chronic infections. Sonoma County, where we live, is rife with CLD and underreported. It is an epidemic of great proportions. It is not understood by the majority of practitioners, and they choose to deny what they don't understand. The primary concern of the director was that it should not matter what brought someone to the ER, but to give them what they need once they are there. The second concern was that the hospital would get a bad reputation in the community because of what I tell anyone who listens about what happens to my daughter in this ER.

Amanda has lost over 100 pounds. She has no more wiggle room. Her body is starved for protein. She has no appetite most of the time due to the nausea. She has to set an alarm clock to take her medicines on schedule or she will begin to throw up. She is in constant pain, even on high doses of narcotics. She would be dead by now if she hadn't had someone who understood her issues and had advocated for her. Every time we start to treat the infections, she gets sicker from the effects of the die-off and toxins. Her immune system is so compromised from the years of untreated infection that it becomes a relentless cycle. Amanda is one of the sickest seen in our practice. Treatment can't be pushed and must be in very small increments. She spends over 50% of her time in bed, often more. Fatigue is a constant.

Amanda's story is not finished. Because she has had these infections for so many years, it will take many years to get better. Amanda has Lyme, Bartonella, Babesia, Chlamydia, and probably, Ehrlichia and Mycoplasma. We haven't tested for viruses because they are low priority. She may have intestinal parasites, and she has been treated for Candida and mold already. The body has to be able to handle the treatment, and without a functioning gut, that can't happen. Amanda avoids dairy, wheat, and soy products as they tend to cause a worsening of symptoms.

Lily, age 11, is Amanda's daughter. She probably has CLD as it passed through the placenta while Amanda was pregnant with her. She gets respiratory infections and other illnesses frequently. She is very labile emotionally. She is defensive and takes things very personally. The family will need to address this soon.

As the mother of a child with CLD, time for my personal life is often placed on hold. I don't work as much as I would like. Sleep is a luxury due to the stress. Our financial resources are depleted. I feel like there is a hammer over my head, ready to drop at any moment. I am working to accept that Amanda may choose to give up. I still hope. I believe healing is possible for her, if she chooses.

As a knowledgeable health care provider and Lyme literate, I find it incomprehensible that the current medical system shuns and marginalizes people with CLD. My daughter's story exemplifies this wrong and shows the need for a place those with CLD can find solace, support, and respect, as well as treatment that moves them toward a healing state.

5: THE DENIAL OF OUR HEALTH CARE SYSTEM

"The intensity of our denial equally mirrors the intensity of our experience."
Anonymous

MICHELE'S STORY

MICHELE CONSIDERS HER PROBLEMS AS "Lyme Light." Michele does not remember being bitten by a tick in the United States, but she went to Africa in 2006 and had six bites simultaneously on her hand. The ticks caused an immediate reaction. Michele experienced significant loss of energy, an aching all over, frequent sweats, and her hand hurt terribly. She tried to take Benadryl, but that didn't work. A few doctors were on the safari, and they didn't know what might be happening. When she got home, she tried to set up an appointment with her "travel doctor." She had another provider look at the bites, but no biopsy was done. The initial reaction eventually went away.

No specific symptoms occurred after that, but then she went to Sri Lanka to work with a small non –profit after the tsunami. When she returned to the United States, tingling and numbness, and restless leg symptoms began. Headaches and pain that was flu-like in nature spread over her body. Then Michele began seeing doctors. She was tested for heavy metals, like mercury and lead, which were elevated. Treatment was done to remove them from her body. Michele saw a rheumatologist who tested for auto-immune diseases, and the results were negative. Michele saw a neurologist, and those results were also negative. She began adjusting her diet and taking supplements. Michele saw as acupuncturist and got massages, but nothing made a difference.

Michele was living in the Los Angeles area during this time. Eventually, she moved to northern California when her mother was diagnosed with lung cancer and needed help. Michele has a sister with CLD, who is now better, and she was too sick to help with their mother's care. Once she moved, the chronic pain started and became severe. A degenerative disc was found in her neck, but the doctors said it was not responsible for the body pain, which was like fibromyalgia. She went to see a naturopathic physician and was placed on several supplements. Again, Michele went through all kinds of tests, which all came back negative. She saw another neurologist and got nowhere. She tried injections, which did nothing. Eventually, Michele had surgery for the disc, which helped somewhat, allowing her to feel healthier. However, the muscle pain did not improve. Inflammation set in and started to affect her daily life. Without energy, she would spend days in bed.

Finally, in July, she saw a Lyme-literate doctor for the first time. Michele was diagnosed with fibromyalgia. Then in January of 2009, she was tested for Lyme at Igenex, a lab in the San Francisco area that comes the closest to getting accurate labs as any lab in the country, but still is not reliable each time. A CD 57 panel was done. A CD 57 panel is a specialized test that measures a specific complement of white blood cells, which helps in determining whether Bb and other co-infections are present and how much they are affecting a person. It can be used to measure progress of treatment, so getting a baseline is a good place to start with the initial evaluation. Michele's level was 48, which indicates exposure to Lyme. A C4a level was elevated. This test measures inflammation. However, the Western Blot for Lyme and the standard test for Lyme were considered negative, even though there was an indeterminate reaction. Over the next few years, Michele continued to have the same symptoms. Then, in January of 2011, her CD 57 panel dropped to 24, and Michele was diagnosed with Lyme. A level this low indicates not only Lyme, but co-infections, as well. Initial treatment was with an herbal tincture, called A-L and made up of many herbs that target Lyme. Later, she was placed on A-Bart, a tincture for Bartonella infection, and now she is taking antibiotics, also. The cost of testing was a burden for her.

She says that without her sister being ill with Lyme, it would have taken her longer to discover her own diagnosis.

Michele says living with a chronic problem has hurt her confidence. She was unable to work for three years because of the pain and loss of energy. Now she is reinventing herself. She has been depressed due to the symptoms. She is terrified she won't be able to work and fearful the pain will stop her progress. She is afraid to talk with people about it. "It feels like this thing that comes between you and life." You lose your life force. For Michele, her life force is coming back slowly. It is so difficult to live this way. She doesn't want it to be the rest of her life. Sometimes the despair is overwhelming. It's all about quality of life and trying your best, but then it becomes unbearable at times. She used to sing and paint but has stopped since she became ill. It takes too much energy. She does not pursue a career full time because she doesn't know from day to day how she is going to feel. Michele feels fortunate to have the support of her sister and a partner. Her joy of life has been challenged, but her positive attitude gets her through the rough spots.

People with Chronic Lyme Disease feel terrible. Imagine feeling exhausted most of the time, having no energy. You hurt everywhere, especially in your joints. The pain can be severe. You may be nauseous every waking minute and eating takes effort. Brain fog is persistent, and you cannot concentrate. Headaches are a daily occurrence, with light and sound sensitivity that drives you away from people and into your home. Depression is pervasive, and sometimes ideas of suicide enter your thoughts. Neurological symptoms, such as tingling and numbness, and electrical, painful shocks travel up your arms and legs, coming and going. It is hard to get out of bed in the morning and function in daily life activities.

Besides feeling terrible and having to struggle to get from place to place, you go to one doctor after another who tells you there is nothing wrong because all the test results are negative. Then you are offered an antidepressant because it must be all in your head. Unfortunately, with Lyme disease and its co-infections, because these are bacterial and parasitic infections affecting different parts of the body, antidepressants are usually ineffective.

Later you are sent to some specialist, a rheumatologist or an infectious disease specialist, and these specialists again do testing which is negative; therefore, again it's believed you don't have any disease. Instead of looking at the clinical picture being presented to them, these physicians say there is nothing wrong. It is implied that it is all in your head. Over and over again, this scenario plays out until you feel like you are going crazy.

Family members look at you like you're going insane, and your loved ones begin to turn away from you. However, you remain caught in this horrible cycle of feeling terrible, not being able to function on a daily basis, and being in pain most the time. It is devastating in every which way—physically, emotionally, spiritually, mentally, and financially.

Since insurance will not cover a problem that does not exist, the costs are extremely high. Not only must you pay for a health insurance policy and the attendant co-pays that go with it, you go to doctors who say nothing is wrong. Then you seek out, if you are lucky to find one, a Lyme-literate provider who does not take your insurance. Most Lyme specialists have cash practices because they could not stay in business otherwise. It takes one to two hours at an initial visit to tease out the problems and begin to address them. At your primary doctor's office, you pay your co-pay, the doctor bills your insurance the remainder, and this doctor only spends five to ten minutes with you. How can anyone know what is going on in such a short period of time? It is not possible. Your story, your symptoms, how you live on a daily basis are important in diagnosing your illness and deciding on the first step in treatment. Lyme patients will pay anywhere from $350 to $1,000 for an initial visit.

Treatment can last for years, depending how long you have been ill before having a correct diagnosis. It can involve intravenous antibiotics, which are very, very expensive. It can involve implanting a semi-permanent central line so that you can continue to get antibiotics intravenously, and all of the supportive therapy that goes along with it; for example, a nutritional supplement for liver support so that the liver continues to function, basic vitamins and minerals, immune system enhancers, probiotics to support healthy intestinal flora, binders to remove the toxins and bacterial die off that occurs with treatment, extra B12 to help energy, and Vitamin D.

People with Lyme disease need to be on supportive therapies and need to be consistent in taking them in order to improve their quality of life and get better.

The emotional costs to a patient and their families are horrendous. How does an ill person participate in life? People with CLD are dependent on family and friends to take care of them, to prepare food for them, to do their errands, to pick up their medicines, to call the doctor and arrange for appointments, to help with their children, if they have any—basically any activity healthy people take for granted.

The insurance companies were paying for all the time Amanda spent in the emergency room and in the hospital, but nothing was done to better her, to help her move forward. All they accomplished was to stabilize her and send her home because they wouldn't recognize that she had infectious disease. This is an incredible waste of resources. If only a third of that cost was directed toward treatment that would allow a person to move forward, they would significantly improve. An ER visit is billed at approximately $5,000 for eight hours. For Amanda, that is 14 ER visits or $70,000 billed for rehydration, intravenous medicine, physician supervision, nursing care, labs, and a bed. Time spent was about 112 hours at $625 an hour. This kept her alive, so it is worth it to us, but such a waste to the world. Proactive care costs much less, and our health care system won't pay for that. While Amanda was an inpatient in the hospital, her care costs were significantly higher.

People with CLD are often afraid to seek help outside of the one provider that they've found who understands their illness. When they're really, really sick, a trip to the emergency room becomes vital to their survival; they have to see other doctors to get emergent care, and the doctors often treat them very badly.

One of the consequences of denying that Chronic Lyme Disease exists is that people are misdiagnosed. Based upon the misdiagnosis, they are given medications and other treatments that are in and of themselves very, very expensive and end up doing no good at all for the person.

Actually, the wrong treatment can do significant harm. Many autoimmune diseases, like Multiple Sclerosis, Systemic Lupus Erthymatosis (SLE), and Rheumatoid Arthritis, other forms of arthritis, ALS or Lou Gehrig's disease, SLE or Systemic Lupus

Erthymatosis, and Parkinson's disease, are frequent misdiagnoses. Autoimmune diseases are a category of chronic illnesses that involve the body turning against itself. For example, the body recognizes a protein in the body that is normally present as something that should not be there and attacks it. Often this happens when the intestinal tract becomes more permeable, allowing proteins that normally remain in the intestinal tract to get out into the general circulation.

A Lyme diagnosis should be considered for any neurodegenerative disease, especially if the specialist calls it "atypical." If a Lyme diagnosis is missed and an autoimmune disease diagnosis is given, then the medicines that are prescribed for these issues actually make the CLD worse. They include immune suppressants and potent anti-inflammatories, called steroids that wipe out what little benefit the immune system is giving to a person with CLD. When someone has been infected for 10 to 20 years before an adequate diagnosis is made, and during that time they are given steroids or immune suppressants, they become much sicker and the medicines usually don't allow them to feel better. It is more difficult to treat them as the immune system must be reactivated in a healthy way before any therapy can begin. This takes time.

Chronic Fatigue Syndrome and Fibromyalgia are not a diagnosis that addresses the core problem, but they are frequent misdiagnoses for CLD. They are a constellation of symptoms that are frequently seen, so they have been named, and they are at least recognized by the current health care system as legitimate problems. It took years for Chronic Fatigue and Fibromyalgia to be recognized, and many physicians still fail to accept them as physical, rather than mental, problems. In our practice, many of these patients have been correctly diagnosed with CLD and effectively treated.

Other problems that mimic Lyme disease must be explored. Mold sensitivity is a poison for many people, and all their symptoms will be very similar to CLD. Their joints will hurt, their memory will be poor, and they'll have brain fog and terrible fatigue. They don't feel well, and they have a difficult time. Often Chronic Fatigue syndrome is diagnosed for mold toxicity. Heavy metal toxicity is another problem that mimics Lyme. We are continually exposed to heavy metals throughout our lives. Heavy metals cause similar symptoms, and, like Lyme, they hide in the tissues. If a doctor does a blood test to look for mercury or lead or another heavy metal, the blood serum values will usually be low. If they are elevated or abnormal, that person is really poisoned. Testing for heavy metals is done often by integrative providers. A provoking agent is used to pull the metals out of the tissues, and then they are measured in the urine. If high, this can be treated. Some allergies, parasite infections, fungal infections, and intestinal infections can mimic symptoms of Lyme, so these possibilities need to be eliminated as a possible diagnosis, too.

Lyme disease is a reportable disease to the CDC and local public health agencies. Sometimes when the local public health agency is called, they refuse to take your report because they tell you that it does not exist in their state or county. It doesn't exist because they don't take the reports. I have heard ludicrous statements like, "There are only two known cases of

Lyme in Sonoma County." One of the local support groups has seen over 500 people with CLD. We have thousands in our practice with CLD. This area is riddled with Lyme. Riddled!

In endemic areas like Sonoma County, familial stories that people tell give a clue to the pervasiveness of misdiagnosis. "My mother died of multiple sclerosis or Parkinson's." This person's mother probably had CLD. This is currently happening across the country. Hunters, hikers, animal enthusiasts, and horseback riders are all at risk for having CLD, without even knowing they were bitten by a tick. This lack of awareness is more menacing than ignorance. Since this is a denied illness, the refusal to acknowledge it is hurting millions of people. These infections are transmitted sexually and through blood transfusions. So being a Good Samaritan and donating blood may be causing more disease than it cures. They test for HIV and disallow anyone who is HIV positive to donate blood, but if you have CLD and don't know it, you are giving blood filled with infectious disease to someone, rather than saving their life. And, having an intimate relationship with a person infected with CLD passes the infection to them. Several couples have been treated for CLD.

This epidemic is more widespread than HIV-AIDS, the plague, bird flu virus, and H1N1 combined.

6: BLENDING THE BEST OF BOTH WORLDS

IT IS TIME FOR A new paradigm in health care.

There are many differences between the way Western health care and Eastern health care deal with Lyme disease and other co-infections. While most of the providers who practice in our current system fail to acknowledge CLD, it is often an acupuncturist or naturopathic physician that suggests the possibility of CLD to a person and gets them to begin looking for other providers who understand what they might be going through.

In an integrative practice, the best of both worlds are utilized in a blended way by using herbals, neutraceuticals, and antibiotics. Using nutrients and herbals, instead of drugs, can control many chronic conditions, as they have fewer side effects and are accepted by the body more readily. For example, it is possible to lower blood sugar using a combination of Alpha Lipoic Acid and cinnamon. Lowering cholesterol can be accomplished using sustained release niacin, red yeast rice, and high-grade fish oil. Use of an enzyme like nattokinase and fish oil together are often more effective than using blood thinners and pose less risk of abnormal bleeding. There are several natural anti-inflammatories that include turmeric, boswellia, and fish oil that can reduce pain, as well as inflammation. Likewise, there are herbal tinctures specific to the treatment of Lyme and the co-infections that work well in combination with antibiotics. Other supplements are utilized to help the body clear toxins from the bugs and support the lymph and liver system, for example.

EDUCATION

In terms of educating the public about this serious epidemic, the California Lyme Disease Association and the International Lyme Disease Association are doing what they can to get into schools and educate children. Unfortunately, a huge population of children is ill with these infections. They are outside playing, and they easily pick up a tick or two. Ticks, when they bite you, have an anesthetic in their bite, so they are designed to bite, get what they need from you, and fall off before you even know they are there. With children, this is even more common. Children with emotional problems, children with autism, and children with other diagnoses like bipolar disorder, schizophrenia, or personality disorders need to be evaluated for Lyme disease. Often, all psychological problems will go away when the Lyme disease is addressed.

MY SON'S STORY AS TOLD BY A MOTHER WHO HAS CURED HER LYME DISEASE AND RECOGNIZED THE SYMPTOMS

"The Bite:

Toward the end of April of 2011, my three-year-old son, "Jake," came home from preschool with a tick on his hand. I did not see the tiny, pin-head size tick until after his bath time, as he was getting ready for bed. (Children move so fast; they rarely sit still long enough to be looked at closely. I mention this because it is of particular interest to me to think about how to best address the issue of Lyme infections in children. The needs and requirements are a bit different than for adults.)

My son loves to "work" in the school garden, so there are frequently small scratches or marks on his hands from digging. I saw something quite different on that day and grabbed his little hand. "Let me see that!" I looked and saw a tiny black speck surrounded by a flat, pink disc shaped rash on the back of his hand. It was a very pale pink rash, not raised, and without a ring. However, it was quite different from any other rashes and certainly not like any bug bites. It did not itch or irritate Jake at all.

The Symptoms:

I decided to wait and see if he came down with any symptoms. It would have been smart to save the tick and get it tested; however, I did not think of this at the time. What I thought of is that if this was a Lyme tick, I was going to have a difficult time ahead of me. And I dreaded the notion. Being a Lyme survivor myself, I know full well the difficulty in getting doctors to listen, let alone diagnose or treat you. I prayed it was "nothing" and put it out of my mind. However, within two weeks, something happened that put my denial to rest. I went to check on my son one night and found him sleeping and in a full-body sweat. His head and hair were soaked. His clothes were soaked, and his sheets were soaked. He continued to have night sweats for close to a week. During that time, he was having other "flu-like" symptoms. He was listless, had a low fever intermittently, and was extremely cranky and irritable. He also complained about severe pain in one leg. His overall look was one of exhaustion, with deep, reddish circles under his eyes and a grey complexion. (This is a place, again, where it merits noting the difference in diagnosing children. Small children may not say, "I feel flu-like." They may not tell you about half of their symptoms. Children are cranky at times, so how do you pick out a particular set of symptoms for them? I was alerted by the profuse night sweats and took note quickly of the rest. This is something parents will have to be educated on, so they can look for subtle, but significant, differences in their children's behavior, and even begin to take note of cycles, if they arise.)

I made an appointment to see his doctor at the local clinic. We actually saw a nurse practitioner. I took my mom with us, as I knew I might need an advocate to help me get through to them. After much discussion, the nurse agreed to order the ELISA Lyme test and prescribe Amoxicillin. This sounds effective on the surface, and most parents would not know they were still far away from success. The ELISA test is notoriously inaccurate, producing false negatives routinely. The Amoxicillin prescription was for ten days. The Lyme spirochete must be treated for at least six weeks, in the earliest stages, to eliminate it in all its growth cycles. In ten days, you might kill all of the most active bugs and leave all the immature ones and those still in the "egg" form. This type of inadequate treatment is what leads to the tragic long-term cases you hear about, of Chronic Lyme Disease. Luckily, I knew this.

Testing:

To begin with, I asked the nurse if we could order a more sensitive test independently, from IGenex. She did not know about the lab, but said it was fine with her. Amazingly, for a person who knew what test to take and how to get, it still took weeks to get a valid test for Jake, because we had to fight the system all the way. First, we ordered the test from IGenex. It took about five days to get it in the mail. Then we had to figure out how to get it to the lab. We needed a physician to authorize the test order. We had to go back to the nurse. When we were finally able to see her, she refused. She did not give much of a reason. She felt she had given us a sufficient course of antibiotic and she had done enough. She said she wasn't convinced he even had Lyme. Although she'd prescribed the Elisa blood test and both blood draws could be done at once, she simply refused to order the more sensitive test. It was at this point that I was most appalled. She did not have to do any extra work. The test required no further blood draw, so it posed no further strain on my child, and it would provide the most accurate information available. Didn't my son deserve this? And what was the alternative? This nurse was willing to take a gamble on my son's life. She was willing to guess that he'd be okay. She was willing to guess that he probably didn't have a Lyme infection. She was willing to roll the dice for him. I, however, was not. I was not willing to gamble on him developing severe neurological disorders over the course of his lifetime. I was not willing to gamble on a lifetime of suffering for him: pain, disorientation, cognitive disruption, depression and anxiety, arthritis, chronic fatigue...

Getting help:

I hurried to the one place in the county that I know treats Lyme disease effectively. It is the place where I was treated years ago. Unfortunately, they are very expensive and do not accept any insurance. Being a low-income family, we really cannot afford such places. It was devastating to me to learn that there was no alternative. There was no place in the county where we could go to get Jake effective care, other than this expensive private clinic. I went in person to plead our case. We just needed the test request. Luckily, they were able to get an appointment for us fairly quickly with a nurse practitioner there who specializes in Lyme disease. She met with us the next day and ordered the test and prescribed a proper course of antibiotics for Jake. She was very kind and did her work in short time increments, so our costs were not astronomical. As it is, they were too high for us, but I was willing to pay the price to get Jake treated. It took a full five more days to get him the test, however, because they did not have the capabilities at that clinic to draw blood from a child. We had to make an appointment for him at Quest, and that had to be done early in a week, so they can send out the test to IGenex before week's end. We did this, and started Jake on the Amoxicillin.

Lyme treatment:

Jake did well for a few days on the Amoxicillin. Then his symptoms worsened. This is normal. And it is a good sign that we were on the right track. The reason is that as the bug is killed, the toxins it produces are released into the system and the patient experiences a worsening of symptoms. (One symptom he had was extreme exhaustion in the afternoons. Again, this is a sidebar to note special attention that must be given to kids. An afternoon nap might seem normal for many kids, and doctors might dismiss this. But for Jake, it is not normal at all. He was never a good napper and gave up his "second nap" when he was one year old, when most kids nap two times a day. He gave up his afternoon nap a bit past two. Afternoon napping is NOT normal for him. And the quality of his napping was particularly noteworthy. He would fall into a deep, exhausted, and sound sleep that was nearly impossible to disturb. He would sleep for between 1.5 to 3 hours. This was so uncharacteristic for him; it was obviously related to the disease. Another symptom was that he was unusually wakeful in early mornings, easily awoken, and finding it impossible to go back to sleep. He is normally most sleepy and hard to wake early in the morning, and I saw this as a classic "sleep disturbance" associated with Lyme. But parents must be very aware of their children's normal behavior and variations, or they can easily be dissuaded by those who don't know their kids.)

This increase in symptoms occurs for a time, until the bug is really reduced and the toxin level from "die-off" is less. I felt sure we'd get a positive result on the test. It took almost two more weeks to get those results. It took one week for the lab to return the results to the doctor's office and another week to get an appointment with the nurse we'd seen. She told us

Jake was positive for Lyme. I was not the least surprised. At the writing of this story, Jake has been on Amoxicillin for about a month. I'm seeing a marked improvement. He does not need those afternoon naps any longer and can take a ride in the car in the afternoon without falling asleep. He is sleeping through the night undisturbed. He is not so anxious or hyper in between periods of exhaustion. He is eating better. In general, there is a mellowing of his moods and evening of his behavior. He is not struggling to find words or remember things as much as he was six or eight weeks ago. I am hopeful that with a continued course of healing, addressed by our properly trained and educated physician, the nurse practitioner at the clinic, we will get Jake through these infections and any possible co-infections. I know that my job as his mother will be to stay alert during his lifetime of any residual symptoms, any cyclical symptoms or behaviors or challenges, and to address them quickly. It is my mission to do anything in my power to ensure that my child has a healthy, full childhood, free of disease, no matter what the medical establishment may think! I am not willing to wait for the general public or the state to catch up in their understanding of this devastating disease. I will be doing all I can for my child right now."

Jake is recovering. He is sleeping undisturbed. He no longer requires naps. His appetite has normalized. Jake is laughing and playing again.

Imagine if you are a parent whose child becomes ill, but you do not know about Lyme. You take your child to their pediatrician and nothing is done because they think your child has Attention Deficit Disorder.

Children with emotional problems, children with autism, and children with other diagnoses, like bipolar disorder, schizophrenia, or personality disorders, need to be evaluated for Lyme disease, as there appears to be a close association between Lyme disease and these problems. Most physicians do not consider Lyme. It would be a shame if a youngster had a treatable case (infection for less than a year) and remained untreated for years because no professional had looked. Often, any psychological behavior will go away when the Lyme is treated. It is critical to educate parents and teachers about this constellation of infections to prevent years of illness and disability. I had no clue when Amanda was bitten that we should pursue more investigation. I thought she had emotional problems— that the vomiting and pain were part of the reaction to her trauma. It is wrong. The denial in our health care system is hurting our children and us.

Whatever the reason, and usually it is the money, the politics of CLD impact every person with this diagnosis. Follow the money and you frequently find that those with influence have a vested interest in maintaining the status quo. The American Infectious Disease Association has done the most damage in perpetuating the myth that CLD doesn't exist. I recently had a 39-year-old woman come into the clinic who has been ill for 20 years. She has lived in an area where there were ticks everywhere in the grass. She was an avid hiker. She knows she was exposed to ticks, had more than one tick bite, and once, had a perfect ring rash on her knee, which she documented with photographs. She showed them to her doctor, who said, "Oh, that's nothing." Well, a ring around a tick

bite is a diagnosis of Lyme disease, period! People who
have this reaction need to be on antibiotics for a
minimum two months to avoid the sequential effects
of a chronic, debilitating disease, which this becomes
over time. She was denied appropriate treatment
because of the politics surrounding CLD and the lack
of knowledge pervasive currently in the Western
Health Care System.

A big issue is awareness. Sixty-five percent of the
people who end up with CLD don't even realize they
have been bitten by a tick. It is looking at the clinical
picture that is critical. Going to a provider who
understands the clinical picture, asks the right
questions, and listens to the story is how CLD is
determined. Increasing awareness in the general
population will eventually force the Western Health
Care System to get involved. One of the physicians I
work with once said that it will take a senator or
representative in Washington to step forward and
promote change in the system. A family member of the
senator or someone they know will tell them their
story and express the horrors of finding a real diagnosis
and adequate treatment before this epidemic is given
the attention it deserves. As of this writing, a new bill
has been introduced in the Senate called the Lyme and
Tick-Borne Disease Prevention, Education, and
Research Act. This is very exciting news.

Pearl is a health care professional who has worked
in the Western Health Care System for 30 years. Until
she contracted Lyme disease, she had great respect for
the system. Now she feels it has failed her.

PEARL'S STORY

Pearl was in excellent health in the spring of 2009. She had been swimming, biking, and hiking. Her diet was clean and healthy, and she used nutritional supplements to enhance her well-being. Two days after hiking in the Sonoma Valley, she brushed a tick off of her head. Pearl called an "on-call MD" and had a lab test mailed to her for use six weeks later. Instead of waiting to take the test, she went to her primary doctor to have the site of the bite examined, hoping to get a prescription for an antibiotic at that visit.

Pearl is an RN and has worked in the hospital as a nurse for 30 years. She had spoken with another physician at the hospital where she worked, who told her that if it were her, she would do a prophylactic shot of penicillin derivative within the first 72 hours after the bite. This is what hastened her trip to her doctor, who refused to give the shot.

In July of 2009, Pearl had one positive IgM band, 41, and was told she did not have Lyme exposure. The 41 band is not specific for Lyme; however, having the blood drawn at a regular lab, rather than Igenex, means that her test could have been a false negative. Too many tests are false negatives! No further discussion of other testing was offered to Pearl.

By 2010, she began to experience symptoms of overwhelming stress on her immune system. Several herpes outbreaks occurred. She had sores in her mouth on more than one occasion, which were diagnosed as Jalapeno exposure. In March and April, overwhelming fatigue occurred daily. Headaches in her frontal area started. Pain and numbness in her legs, sweating, overwhelming neck pain, and noticeable skipped beats in her heart would wake her up at night and keep her awake. Pearl thought she might have a cold or flu, and sinus issues. She tried Claritin without any benefit. Pearl attributed the heart symptoms to stress and the neck pain to needing a chiropractic adjustment. Other random pains and symptoms kept happening.

The cardiac pains were particularly alarming—often she would experience air hunger or shortness of breath. As a nurse, she knew something was not right with her cardiac function. Fatigue continued to worsen, and it became difficult to muster the energy to get out of bed in the morning. She would wake up poorly refreshed and would drag herself out of bed, drink coffee, and drag herself to work. At the end of the day, once back home, she would lie on the couch without the energy to make herself dinner. In May, several episodes of radiating arm pain accompanied by severe, piercing chest pain, neck pain, and jaw pain frightened her terribly. Pearl had no doubt that these symptoms were heart related. She would try to decrease her stress level and rest with episodes of pain. Finally, after several bouts of pain, she disclosed her symptoms to her nurse co-workers who sent her immediately to the ER. She was relieved of her duties.

The ER report indicated ectopic beats or irregular beats and first degree heart block. She was sent immediately to a cardiologist. The cardiology workup did not indicate coronary artery disease, so the situation was attributed to stress. Pearl then took the rest of the summer off to de-stress. By the end of the summer, Pearl had pain in every joint of her body, no resolution of her heart symptoms, and cognitive problems and memory loss, so seeking work as a nurse became unrealistic.

At the prompting of a friend, Pearl sought more testing for arthritis and Lyme. The doctor she saw wanted to diagnose her condition as Chronic Fatigue Syndrome and Fibromyalgia.

"Night terrors" was another diagnosis which was due to Pearl admitting she had a dream about Spirochetes. Pearl has prophetic dreams and is an instructor of dream interpretation. In fact, she has had several dreams which have guided her in seeking treatment for her CLD. However, Lyme has affected her ability to dream. She was planning to teach a course in dream interpretation before she became ill. The infection is in her temporal lobe, and this interferes with picture recognition. In June of 2010, Pearl had a dream about Spirochetes before she tested positive for Lyme. She had another dream about parasites. She saw a lot of parasites. In August of 2010, also before diagnosis, she saw a group of people sitting together and reading official books in another dream. She went away, and when she came back, they were all dead from a poison that killed them simultaneously. She felt that some of the people were trying to see what had happened and understand it. She saw a prophetic woman who was being blamed, but it wasn't her fault. Pearl sees herself as this woman. "Why is this massacre happening?" It is a metaphor for what is occurring in the WHCS that denies everything about Lyme. The CLD patient is constantly marginalized, blamed, told they are crazy, yelled at, refused care, and their reality is denied. People are dying from CLD that is going undiagnosed and untreated!

More testing was done through Igenex lab that showed a positive Lyme and Babesia test. Pearl finally had proof of her illness. She was given 28 days of Doxycycline. As Pearl was researching her condition, she realized her level of illness required more than this one drug—and for a longer period of time. After several visits to different specialists who all refused to treat her, Pearl sought the expertise of a Lyme–literate holistic provider. A CD 57 panel was done that showed Lyme. "In network" physicians have been less than helpful, creating intense frustration, grief, and shock. She tried to get IV antibiotics and Mepron for the Babesia infection. Repeatedly, these doctors insinuated that people with psych diagnoses run from doctor to doctor, thinking they have Lyme disease. Isn't this convenient? Meanwhile, Pearl and others like her are struggling physically with an illness and not receiving proper treatment.

Pearl went on disability and is paying hundreds of dollars for health insurance so she can retain the ability to keep insured without a pre-existing condition. As a nurse in the WHCS, Pearl has repeatedly attempted to get her network physicians to render treatment to her so insurance will pay. They have all refused. An infectious disease physician at UCSF initially told her to get on IV Rocefin, and then changed his mind three days later. She is furious and outraged by the systematic way her diagnosis has been ignored, her logical questions have been overridden, and the pattern that is being established in her medical record that it is all in her head. This is truly negligence.

Pearl again visited the Lyme-literate provider in December 2010 and was given the appropriate medicines for treating Babesia, as well as an herb that helps to get at the parasite. She tried to stop the doxycycline, but brain issues returned and she went back on it. Currently, Pearl is on IV Rocefin, which gets at most of the bacterial infections, including Lyme, Bartonella, Ehrlichia, and Mycoplasma. She has some days that are good, and she can function better at times. Her story continues. Pearl has a positive psychological outlook, despite what she has experienced in trying to get treatment. She has done a lot of spiritual work and feels she got this illness so she could bring it to the light and help others. This will do more for a cure than almost anything else. Without strong mental health, it is not possible to get better.

Thora is another victim. She got better and is now an advocate for those dealing with CLD and actively involved with the California Lyme Disease Association. She has been working for years to increase awareness and improve access to care. Thora has helped so many. When I speak to almost anyone in the Sonoma's "Lyme community," I hear her name.

THORA'S STORY

This tale begins back in 1988 when Thora was ill with an odd assortment of distressing symptoms. She went to 12 different physicians in seven months and was diagnosed with many problems, from stress-related disorders to encephalitis. She had severe pain and anxiety and was distraught with the uncertainty of what was happening to her. In October, she was finally told she had Lyme disease. Thora began treatment immediately.

In April of 1988, April had been walking and hiking in the Sonoma hills. Two weeks after hiking, Thora developed a bull's eye rash on her neck. This is diagnostic of active Lyme disease. She went to her doctor, who gave her a cream to put on the hot and itching rash. Next came a stiff neck and shooting pains in her left arm, then the stabbing, shooting pains moved to her right leg and her right foot began to feel numb. This indicates a Bartonella infection. Memory loss followed.

Thora was a supervisor in an accounting office. Her co-workers began telling her more and more that she wasn't remembering discussions and decisions. She began to write notes to remind her of issues and then would lose the notes. She demoted herself to a bookkeeper.

The pain grew worse. She forgot what her car looked like. It was frightening for her. Her next step was to see a neurologist, who told her he was considering the possibility that she had Multiple Sclerosis and brain tumors. An MRI was ordered. All lab work was negative, and her condition was labelled stress induced. The neurologist referred her to a psychologist. The suggestion that it was all in her head was insulting, but she went anyway. During the session, Thora began to experience severe heat in her hands and tingling in her legs. Her knees and other joints felt like they were on fire. This sent her flying back to her doctor.

She found the texture of her hands was changing, and they were turning shades of blue, purple, and white. This event was diagnosed as Carpal Tunnel syndrome, so back to the neurologist Thora went. An

MRI of her neck was done, and she was sent to a neurosurgeon to relive the pressure on her vertebrae in her neck. Then, the left side of her face went numb. Another diagnosis was bone spurs, which were treated with cortisone, a potent steroid. The steroid made her worse, her symptoms flared to the point where she could barely walk. Thora was in severe pain but continued to refuse narcotics to relieve it.

After so many diagnoses, her friends and doctors seemed to stop believing her. She knew something was wrong with her—that she was very ill. She was starting to lose the use of her legs. Finally, she asked her doctor to send her to Stanford. This really messed her up. At Stanford, she was told she had viral encephalitis and that she did not have Lyme disease. She asked to see a Lyme specialist, and he told her that Lyme was a fashionable disease that she did not have and gave her Premarin. Needless to say, she left Stanford still ill, frustrated, and very angry. Finally, someone put her on Doxycycline, an antibiotic that treats the Lyme bug, but not the co-infections of Bartonella and Babesia. She stayed on the Doxycycline for a month, and her symptoms improved slightly, but once the month ended, her symptoms returned. The exhaustion and pain were terrible.

Getting nowhere, Thora decided to do her own research on Lyme disease. She discovered that all her symptoms fit Lyme. She began to correspond with the Lyme Borreliosis Foundation in Lyme, Connecticut, where the first outbreak of Lyme was detected in 1975, and she found a Lyme support group in Ukiah. At the support group, Thora was advised to go back on antibiotics. Thora was in intense pain, and the pain in her elbows made her feel like they were broken. Her feet hurt more than ever.

Her next stop was to see an infectious disease physician in Santa Rosa who confirmed that she did have Lyme disease. She received IV antibiotics for only two weeks and then spent the next year on oral antibiotics. This helped her to get her life back.

Over the years, she has intermittently taken more antibiotics. She has more energy, but still tires easily and must pace her activities with rest.

Again, with this constellation of infections, it is completely about awareness. If you choose to see your primary provider, then ask them questions such as, "Do you believe that Chronic Lyme Disease exists?" and "What do you think about Lyme disease?" If they respond by saying it doesn't exist, I'd thank them, turn around, and walk out the door. Unfortunately, most people don't do this.

7: DIAGNOSIS

DIAGNOSIS OF CLD IS IN the patient's history.

Testing currently available is inaccurate and unreliable with too many false negatives. The tests are not specific or sensitive enough. Some labs are working diligently to change this and make testing more worthwhile. In addition, the tests cost hundreds of dollars, and the insurance companies won't pay for the tests because they don't believe that there's a problem to begin with, so it comes out of the patient's pocket. Most doctors in the current health care system are accustomed to being able to test for something, and get an accurate positive or negative response on the test. They want a nice, what I call "in the box" formula for diagnosing and treating a problem. "You have pneumonia. Well, we'll put you on an antibiotic for two weeks, and you'll get better." These infections are complex, and each person responds uniquely to their own set of issues, so it is very important to have a close working relationship with a provider who understands how to diagnose and treat them.

In an integrative practice, one way we confirm a probable diagnosis of Lyme is to use herbal tinctures to do what are called challenges. The herbal tinctures are specific to different infections: Bartonella, Babesia, Lyme, etc. If a person is infected with the co-infection being tested, he/she will usually react with an exacerbation of symptoms. This suggests a diagnosis that co-infection is likely. Once a person reacts to the tincture, then it is stopped until the reaction subsides. Treatment begins using a smaller amount of the tincture than was used in the provocation test, which means going very slowly, building up the dose of the tincture. An intense reaction may deter someone from continuing treatment, as it is often worse than the symptoms experienced with the disease. Finding a dosage that will be effective without producing a reaction is suggested.

When somebody reacts really quickly, it's also an indication that their body isn't able to process the toxins that the bacteria is putting out. When the bugs begin to die-off, the body isn't able to get rid of them. It's really important that the body be able to detoxify, to process all of the die-off and toxins and get them out of the body, because if you leave the neurotoxins in the system, they just continue to circulate. Then the problem gets more and more intense, instead of better.

This is why a healthy detoxification response is so important. There are some excellent lab tests that can measure how well a person is able to detoxify, but, again, they are very expensive. If it is necessary to cut costs for a patient, which, of course, they want you to do, challenges are done, along with giving supportive supplements, which help the body through treatment.

MARILYN AND JOHN'S STORY

Marilyn and John grew up in the Sonoma Valley of the Moon. They used to hike and play as children, and as adults, they camped with their family. As a child, Marilyn had to stop playing the piano when she was 13 because of pain and stiffness in her hands and fingers. She had jaw and teeth problems. Headaches were horrible and frequent. Certain foods would cause vomiting. This started when she was 8 years old. At age 18, Marilyn started spitting up blood every morning. This did not stop until she was 34.

It wasn't until 1981 that the real problems began. It felt like the end because no one knew anything. The family was camping on Lake Alminore in their new trailer when Marilyn came down with a high fever and horrific headache. It felt like her brain would explode. This lasted for three days. She sought medical help, telling her doctor that something was very wrong. She was throwing up every day and had severe nausea constantly. Eventually cysts were found in her spleen. When she was 34, her spleen was removed. Before that, she felt like she was walking around with an elephant in her stomach. After the surgery, the elephant was gone. Cysts and multiple lesions were found in her spleen, which was four times larger than a normal spleen. Marilyn did well for two years after; she had more energy for the first time since childhood.

Then in June 1983, she became ill with the flu. She had headache and a fever. From that point on, a low-grade fever was persistent. She was plagued by horrible headaches. Fatigue and joint pain were constant. The next step took her to an infectious disease specialist in Napa, who she saw for a year. They took her uterus when a CT scan showed infection, endometriosis, and an inflamed appendix. She felt he was done with her then. From 1983 until 1989, her problems continued. She visited numerous physicians, including a neurologist, rheumatologist, and another infectious disease doctor and got no help. Walking was difficult in 1989. One day when getting ready for work, she fell and couldn't get back up. Marilyn called her mother, who called the infectious disease physician in Napa, and they went to see him. Marilyn was hospitalized while another barrage of tests was done. At this time, she presented the idea of Lyme disease to the doctor, who told her it did not exist. Despite his response, he gave her an antibiotic for two months. A friend with Lyme disease took her to another physician in Lake County, who treated patients with CLD. After that, she found a doctor in Sonoma who treated Lyme. He gave her an antibiotic called Biaxin, which was a miracle to her. Her memory was awful, and she had to give up reading. Then a six-week run of IV Rocefin was given, but this is not an adequate dose. It is needed for at least three to six months.

Marilyn's husband, John, began to have symptoms in 1989. He also went to several doctors and felt the Biaxin was the best antibiotic he had tried. John had positive tests for Lyme and Babesia and was able to get treatment that was covered by insurance. A rheumatologist he saw gave him fiber for the diarrhea caused by the medicine for Babesia. John spent years on the medicines. He retired in 1993. After, he did chelation for a few years due to cardiac and vascular problems, including leg pain, and this took away the pain in his legs. Eventually, he had bypass surgery on his heart. Babesia causes heart damage. Bartonella causes inflammation in the vascular system. It is possible, in my opinion, that Babesia and Bartonella may have contributed to the need for his surgery.

John is still not sure the infections are gone. He has days when he is down, with no energy. He feels achy and flu-like. He has joint pain daily. Bartonella has not been addressed yet. The tests for Bartonella are almost always negative, even when the clinical picture says otherwise.

For Marilyn, her daily life consists of pain everywhere in her body. The bottom of her feet hurt all the time. Poor energy plagues her on a daily basis. Fortunately, she has no more nausea. She says she would have given up a long time ago were it not for her positive attitude. She probably has Bartonella infection, which has never been addressed. Her most recent CD 57 panel is very low at 30, despite Igenex testing that came back negative for infection. Marilyn's clinical picture is typical of a person with CLD. This should be what drives her treatment, not the testing.

Marilyn finally did an herbal challenge for Bartonella. She reacted after the first dose. This is diagnostic of active infection with Bartonella, and gives information on how sensitive her body has become. Use of a binder, probiotic, and liver support are critical while she begins antibiotics once again. Eventually, Marilyn may need to receive antibiotics for a period of 6 to 12 months to resolve the Bartonella infection.

8: WHAT IS HEALING?

"True healing elicits response from depths of the human condition that are not well understood in our time. Healing aligns with life-affirming forces such as compassion and humane support."
Delores Krieger, PhD., R.N.

HEALING INVOLVES FINDING THE ROOT cause of a problem and then addressing it.

You cannot heal a problem until you know what it is, and that's where Western medicine and integrative medicine go their separate ways. Western medicine takes things and reduces it down to its smallest denominator. "Oh, you have a urinary tract infection. Let's give you an antibiotic," instead of looking at the complete picture, what a person is expressing, and seeing from this what the root of the problem could be, which is what an integrative practitioner does. Then once the root cause or causes are discovered, an integrative provider works along with that person to discover the best way to peel all the layers of the infections away, like peeling an onion. The body tells us where to go by what symptoms are currently bothering the patient most. What they tell you is the most important problem that they're having. For some people, it could be depression, and for others, it could be joint pain. For some, it could be stomach pain.

Whatever they're saying is their biggest priority, and what the practitioner picks up in the clinical picture is where you begin. It's very difficult to treat all of these co-infections at the same time.

Ten to twenty years ago, providers would give antibiotics to patients with Lyme disease. They didn't understand about detoxifying and the metabolic dysregulation that Lyme disease causes. They didn't understand about the hormonal dysregulation that occurs with chronic illness.

Now, it's this big picture of looking at, "Is the thyroid functioning? Are the adrenal glands functioning? Are their sexual hormones at optimal levels?" This is critical because the hormonal system is one key to a high quality of life. "How is their intestinal tract doing? How well do they digest?"

"Do they need to eliminate wheat or gluten, and soy and dairy, or any other foods that they might be sensitive to?" Because when you're sensitive to something like wheat, it creates more inflammation. It is so important to decrease the inflammation in the body at the same time as addressing what the body needs by way of treatment.

For some people, that might be Bartonella. Typically, we look at the co-infections before we go after the Lyme, but with some people, the Lyme is so dominant that that's where to go first. That's where the complexity comes in, and that's where the individualization comes in with each person.

TERESA'S STORY

Teresa is a Registered Nurse. This story is in her words.

"I remember my first tick bite well. It was 1972—spring semester at Chico State, and I was standing across from my Anatomy lab partner, staring at the rock-hard, rangy, formaldehyde-filled cat that we were dissecting. All morning, I had been noticing achy lymph nodes in my left axilla, and during lab, I mindlessly traced the aching to a floppy thing attached under my left breast. Luckily, my lab partner, Sharon, who had grown up in the valleys below Mt. Lassen, knew ticks well and easily removed it, tossing it out after turning it over several times in her hand. In February of '72, I had moved into the Paradise/Magalia area, a community in the foothills of the Sierras. We lived on the side of a canyon, covered in Manzanita, Toyon, Scrub and Ponderosa pines. Our dogs and cat ran freely and carried a lot of ticks into our house. We didn't think twice about them, as we pulled them off our dogs and listened to their sizzling when we threw them into our wood stove.

Two to three weeks later, I developed a red bump on the back of my right thigh. It felt a little achy, and I was concerned enough that I went to the student health center on campus to have it checked out. The doctor told me it was a spider bite and sent me on my way. Over the next several days, a circular rash developed and grew to about 5 inches in diameter. It was a little bumpy around the perimeter, but otherwise flat. It continued to ache a little, and I remember feeling a little flu-like. It did not itch, but I thought perhaps this was my first exposure to poison oak. The episode resolved after a couple weeks and never flared up again.

In the early 80's, I had another tick bite. By early 1982, I was having severe headaches often enough that I went to a neurologist. After a normal CT scan, I was subsequently diagnosed with a combo of muscle tension and migraine headaches. I was a runner, racquet ball player, and taught aerobic dance. From the 80's to the 90's, I experienced migrating joint pain: first my knee, then my ankle, then my elbow or shoulder. None of it was incapacitating, although the headaches seemed to control my life, occurring at least 4 to 5 times a week. I spent a lot of money and time seeking traditional and non-traditional approaches to managing the headaches.

In 1998, I noticed my legs felt achy much of the time while sitting at my desk at work. I described it as a migraine of the body. Over the next couple years, I developed irritable bowel and esophageal reflux and lost weight without trying. There was a fair amount of stress in my life at the time, so the depression and anxiety I was feeling was no surprise. In 2000, recurrent latent herpes infection stemming from childhood exploded, so I started on antivirals and pain medication. Also during that year, waves of tingling – pins and needles – would traverse from my mouth to my fingertips and chest. I underwent two surgeries for a herniated lumbar disk in 2001. In mid-March, 2002, I took two rounds of antibiotics for a particularly stubborn upper respiratory infection. In early April, my equilibrium became altered; I tingled from head to fingertips; I felt disconnected from my body; and I was having vividly freakish nightmares and what seemed to be hallucinations. I was so frightened between 3 and 5 in the morning that I had my husband sit with me to keep me grounded in reality. I continued going to work, although it felt like an out-of-body experience. I remember asking my nurse colleagues for a meeting so I could explain to them what was going on. They were baffled, as was I.

By the end of April, I was having overwhelming head, neck, and upper back pain which radiated into my right shoulder, arm, wrist and hand. It generalized to my left side, also. It was a burning pain that did not respond to analgesics or narcotics. My fingers ached terribly. Aching pain affected my legs, ankles, and feet, which made standing in the kitchen to prepare meals an excruciating and dreaded experience. I was having anxiety and panic attacks. Throughout the following months, I had what seemed to be spasms of consciousness, which felt like what I would expect seizures to feel like. I developed a dry cough. I was nauseated and subsequently lost 23 pounds over the next year. Oddly, I was not necessarily fatigued. However, I could no longer sit at my desk in an upright position and work a full day due to the pain, so I went on partial disability for the next year. Even half-days were too much, although I managed to get through it.

I was under the care of a rheumatologist. Both he and my primary health care provider surmised I had fibromyalgia, although I did not have the typical tender points. My back surgeries in 2001 and the probability that I was peri-menopausal complicated the picture. Yet a woman whom I had gotten to know at a physical therapy pool was convinced my symptoms were consistent with Lyme disease. She was very familiar with Lyme disease because her husband had been recently severely disabled with it after having tick bite on the job as a lineman with PG&E.

I was also under the care of a naturopathic physician/chiropractor who agreed to order the recommended lab work for Lyme and other TBDs through Igenex. In June/2002, my IgM Western Blot came back negative, my IgG was positive, Babesia microti was negative, and the HME (Ehrlichia/Anaplasma) panel indicated past treatment or disease state. I dropped off the lab reports with my primary health care provider; however, she was out of town so another doctor looked at it and pronounced it negative, as I believe she would have, also. Few doctors knew how to read or comprehend the test results then.

I tried multiple times to contact a Bay Area physician with experience with CLD, but could never get through to a live person. He did not respond to my emails. For the next couple years, I vacillated between doing online searches about Lyme disease and trying to forget about the fact that I probably had it and could not get someone to treat me for it. In winter, 2004, I found the name of an infectious disease specialist in Napa on a website about C LD. I made an appointment with him. He ran tests through Quest, and all were negative. Nevertheless, he willingly put me on a month of doxycycline (half the now-recommended dose). My symptoms did not improve, so he concluded that I did not have Lyme disease. By fall of 2005, my rheumatologist diagnosed me with atypical rheumatoid arthritis (RA), as labs such as rheumatoid factor and C-reactive protein were always negative. I had no swelling in my joints. I started treatment for RA, which soon included Placquenil and weekly Methotrexate (MTX) injections. I would get an injection on Thursday afternoon, and on Saturday, I would be bedridden with pain and fatigue (in retrospect, probably a Herxheimer reaction). I would recover on Sunday and return to work on Monday. For about a month in spring of 2006, I had a glimpse of normalcy. However, my white blood cell count dropped secondary to the MTX; I experienced two severe respiratory infections and had to go off the MTX.

My primary health care provider did not know what to do with me. I was often desperate and crying during my visits with her. She was not convinced that RA was the correct diagnosis. My pain was so incapacitating that I started using Fentanyl patches, similar to Morphine, first 25 mcg, then 50 mcg, supplementing with Norco for break-through pain and Celebrex, a potent non-steroidal anti-inflammatory. It improved my life greatly, and I felt I could finally look forward to taking part in activities. Among some of the most emotionally stressful issues were getting up each day and making it through a work day, not knowing if I could commit to extracurricular plans, and finding the energy to enjoy my children and young grandchildren.

Once more, I tried medication for RA. I started Enbrel, an immune suppressant, in Sept of 2006 and finally went off it in early 2007 when it did not seem to be helping at all. At that point, I was tired of and actually humiliated by all the doctor- and health care practitioner-shopping, so I just trusted that sooner or later, the right person would enter my path.

In summer of 2008, two things happened. First, I was ready to hit this head on and really know what my symptoms were. So with the help of my primary MD, I tapered off the Fentanyl patches, substituting them with fairly high doses of Norco, which I gradually tapered. However, my inflammation was so extreme that I had to double my Celebrex dose. Second, a colleague of mine shared Dr. H's name with me, describing her as a physician who thought "outside the box." I saw her for the first time in Sept., 2008 at her office in Napa. She listened to my story with interest, took my history, looked at my previous labs, and examined the data like a CSI physician. I was absolutely amazed, gratified, and validated. She felt fairly certain that my diagnosis was surely Lyme and probably another tick-borne disease, but she drew blood again, sent it off to Igenex, and referred me to a Lyme-literate MD closer to where I lived.

By the third week of October, 2008, I had my labs back. My Western Blots, both IgG and IgM, were positive both according to Igenex and CDC/NYS criteria. My test for Babesia duncani was suggestive of infection. My only other result which looked borderline positive was the human granulocytic panel. I met with Dr. M in Sacramento. He felt there was no question that I had Lyme – active Lyme. I started on doxycycline and seemed to HERX for an entire month!! Tingling, muscle cramping, horrible headaches, dizziness, memory dysfunction, pain, out of body sensation all flooded back again. After one month of apparent Herxheimer reaction, Dr. M suspected that

Babesia needed to be addressed before making headway on the Lyme. Therefore, he discontinued the doxy and started me on the antimalarials, artimisinin and Mepron, plus Azithromycin and Placquenil to continue treating the Lyme. By the end of December, I was flattened with fatigue like I had never experienced before, except during bouts with influenza. I felt toxic and in pain. I realized at this point that I was now being dragged through the tunnel backwards. I knew there was light at the end of the tunnel, but there were so many curves ahead that the light was not visible. I can say that I simply endured through this time, which went on for several months and lessened so very gradually. This "bottoming-out" made very clear how sick I had been. However, I knew I was getting better. As early as January, 2009, I went off my Lexapro, an antidepressant, and have not been on it since. The pain in my lower legs and feet vanished, and the wrist pain lessened gradually. I joined a Pilates class in May of 2009 (with some ups and downs), but overall it was very encouraging.

My medication list was already long. I came to Dr. M on several supplements, like magnesium to treat the twitching and muscle cramping, ferrous sulfate for recently diagnosed anemia and very low iron stores, and some hormones. Dr. H and Dr. M additionally supplemented my treatment over time by addressing all my depleted systems, adding more support with Vitamin B-12, probiotics, Vitamin D, proteolytic enzymes, and chelation therapy. I feel the supplementary support helped bring my body back up to where it could respond well to the antibiotics and antimalarials. Over the span of my 18-24 months of treatment, I took several different antibiotics and antimalarials to treat the different forms of B. burgdorferi and also B. duncani. The antimalarial treatment, I feel, was the turning point for me.

It was such a long journey, yet by one year later, I was feeling so much better. One gauge I used was the level of trepidation I experienced in making future plans. After a year, I had almost forgotten to worry if I would or would not be up to committing to an activity on the weekend.

In the years before treatment, I leaned heavily on my spirituality, and secondly, on my family and select friends, including my cranial-sacral therapist who was a miracle worker. My healing was already taking place before I started actual treatment because I knew someday I would find the right practitioner to walk me through this. However, I feel being a registered nurse was actually a detriment in this situation because I dreaded going to doctors during that pre-treatment period, feeling like I was weak and begging for help. I can certainly advocate for others, but when it came to my situation, I felt very confused.

Presently, 2 ½ years after starting treatment and taking my last Malarone in 12/2010, I feel I am Lyme-free and Babesia-free. I find that my recovery after strenuous or tiring activities and stressful events is slower than I want it to be, and I need to pace myself. I continue to experience some generalized body pain, but how much is due to my back issues, I don't know. Ensuring good sleep is crucial.

I am so very grateful to Dr. M and Dr. H for their brilliant care, as well as my primary physician Dr. N for sticking with me and not referring me to a psychiatrist. My experience has touched many others close to me and in my community, leading others to find much-needed medical treatment. I feel that every person with Lyme disease and other TBDs who are under the care of Lyme-literate health practitioners can be the spark to the healing of so many more individuals who are suffering. It is very gratifying to be able to support others on their way to healing and wellness."

Part of Teresa's story is about being placed on an immune suppressant, Enbrel, which made her symptoms worse. By trying this medication, it made getting to a cure more difficult and lengthened her treatment. This is part of the overall picture of CLD when it is ignored. More harm can be done than good.

The next story is one of hope and surmounting dramatic odds to become well. Linda is a true Lyme Warrior. She has devoted her life to helping others with the disease and is passionate about this work. Linda is convincing when she talks about how to protect yourself from infection. She reminds people to "stay on the asphalt; keep to wide hiking trails; check yourself and your kids for ticks every time you come inside." She adds, "Woman to woman, it's a real dumb idea to seek privacy in the high weeds just because you don't like the trailside convenience."

LINDA'S STORY

Linda was first infected in May, 1989. Before that time, she built bridges and freeways in the San Francisco Bay area. Many told her she was the strongest woman they had ever known. All that changed when she was working as a surveyor tech for a private company near an old vineyard. She came out into a clearing, checked her clothing, and found several ticks. She developed a bull's eye rash on her left hip within three days of the bites. She thought it was a rash caused by friction from carrying her tool pouch. The shadow of the rash lasted eight months.

Then the symptoms started with a stiff neck, sore throat, and headache. She took eight aspirins per day. Linda continued working through the heat of the summer in the central valley. One day, she had severe chest pain and thought she was having a heart attack. She finished work and went to an ER. She found herself getting lost everywhere she went, both in her house and in the town where she lived. Linda got progressively sicker throughout the summer. During this time, Linda was looking for answers to her symptoms and figured she probably had Lyme. She went to a rheumatologist, who told her she didn't have Lyme. However, she did get a two-week prescription for Doxy. She continued working and got blisters under her thumb nails from sun exposure. She didn't notice any change from the medicine.

She got sicker and sicker and stopped working sometime around the end of August. As the symptoms progressed, she got lost at the local grocery store and two friends stepped in to take care of her. At that time, Linda owned five buildings and could no longer take care of or pay for them, so she had to abandon them. She couldn't fill out paper work. With help, she filed for workers' compensation and was granted temporary disability and treatment after the first of the year. The disability lasted for a few years. Then Linda met Thora, who had gone public with her diagnosis of Lyme, and found a support group, as well as a Lyme-literate MD. Linda feels Thora saved her life by going public.

After two weeks of IV Rocefin, she didn't notice much improvement. Then she went on large doses of Amoxicillin, which also didn't help. She developed Bell's palsy and felt she was detached from the world (Babesia was later diagnosed). She had terrible sweats and nodules under the skin over her neck (lymph glands swollen). Doxycycline became her savior.

She wasn't getting better fast. She couldn't use her mouth for expression due to the Bell's palsy, which took two years to resolve. Linda tested positive on a urine test for Lyme, which helped to keep her disability case open. Linda saw a few providers who specialized in Lyme, and found them to be very helpful. One of them wrote a letter stating that she had a 100% disability. In 1997, a judge overturned her disability case and denied further support. Eventually, she prevailed on appeal and got full disability.

During this time, Linda was living in her car, so it was difficult for her to follow through on the case. She was unable to live in conventional housing due to electrical sensitivity (EMF), which made her sick. She still cannot tolerate EMF and now has emptied her home of this kind of stimulation. Exposure to EMF can stimulate the Lyme bug to move faster. Linda stayed in various state and regional parks in her car for two years.

Finally, Linda found a place with an elderly woman, where she stayed for six months. Then she spent seven years in a camper with no electricity or heat or running water. There were times that icicles froze on the windows. She did, however, have a telephone. She had to use the house bathroom, and the walk to the house was exhausting. She used propane gas to heat water and an icebox to keep food cold. During this period of time, she applied for and got a housing voucher. Today, Linda is living in federally subsidized housing. She turns off many of the circuit breakers to keep the EMF low. Her home has gas heat and a gas stove, which causes less sensitivity than electricity. Her P G & E bill averages a mere $5.00.

While living in the camper, she saw another Lyme literate doctor who diagnosed and treated Babesia. She also got H. pylori and was treated and cured. Her GI tract healed after that. Over all of those years, Linda learned which foods trigger increased symptoms and avoids them. After spending 16 years on different antibiotics, Linda finally stopped taking them six years ago. Her symptoms went away. Now she is hiking and riding a bike. She got her brain back, the Bell's palsy is gone, and pain is rare. EMF or processed foods still trigger headaches, though, and she still has difficulty organizing paper work and mailing letters. She will drive and deliver her bills so they get where they need to be. Her laptop makes her sick, so she seldom uses it.

Linda leads a support group for Lyme patients. About 1 ½ years ago, the group started with six people and now meets weekly. The group is growing, with over 500 people joining in the last year. Linda lobbies to the city council in Sebastopol, Vector Control for Marin and Sonoma counties, and Palm Drive Hospital to urge better awareness and treatment for Lyme.

Linda feels extremely grateful for all the support and help she has had from providers, friends, and others who helped her to get the treatment and dollars to live and get well.

MIND-BODY-SPIRIT-ENERGETIC INTEGRATION

"Pythagoras said that the most divine art was that of healing. And if the healing art is most divine, it must occupy itself with the soul, as well as with the body; for no creature can be sound so long as the higher part in it is sickly."
Apollonius of Tyana

"To release the past, we must be willing to forgive. All disease comes from a state of unforgiveness"
Louise L. Hay

As people, we are not just bodies. We have emotions. We think. We also are spiritual beings. We have a soul. We have energetic bodies that surround our physical body, and all of these things play into how well we are, what kind of quality of life we have, and balancing not just the body.

Dora Kunz believes that, "Illness is disharmony in the organizing patterns of the body. This may take place at different levels. It involves not only the physical damage to the organism but if we think of man as an integrated system, it affects feeling, thinking, and other levels. There is also a spiritual component in each person."

All disease, dis-ease, is really a surface issue. A lot of providers in Western medicine look at cancer, I mean, the results of cancer, that cancer causes changes in the cells. "Oh, these infections or this cancer are intercellular. They get into the cell," which sounds really, really deep in the body.

If one shifts their perception and sees these infections or cancer, or whatever it is that is being addressed, as a surface issue to that person, then that person is not that disease. That person is not cancer. That person is not Lyme disease. But, that person is one of complexity. By addressing mental and emotional attitude, and addressing any trauma, and healing it, the door to healing the infection opens. Counseling becomes an important key to successful treatment. If post-traumatic stress disorder symptoms are present, which frequently are with people with Lyme disease, it needs to be addressed. Every person that I've interviewed as a provider, without exception, has had some form of trauma. The trauma begins to rule their life and affects every decision they make. It's really important for them to shift their perception of the world, to one that's more positive, that gives them an opportunity to think they could feel good, and get well again because if they don't have that, they won't get well. They have to have it. Illness is a message to change. Everyone has his cancer, whether emotional or physical. The person is left with the choice to change and heal, or see their illness as a catastrophe or death sentence. The illness needs to be seen as a message to redirect their life, and, within this transformation, healing happens.

Lyme and the co-infections will cause previous psychological patterns to intensify or cause new patterns to emerge. EMDR, an eye movement therapy that allows access to both sides of the brain at once; EFT or emotional frequency release, which allows a person to work on themselves; journey work; cognitive processing therapy; stress reduction; yoga; and tai chi are some examples that can be helpful for working through these issues. Besides therapy, having strong support from family and friends is very important. If a person is too sick to do anything, then simply sitting out in nature is helpful. Hugging a tree can help to dissipate negative energy. The Chinese believe that if you hug a tree, it will absorb all negativity and anger from your body.

Energetic supportive therapies can be utilized. There's one called Frequency Specific Microcurrent that specifically targets tissues with energy with specific conditions. There's acupuncture and cranial-sacral therapy. Therapeutic touch works on the energy fields surrounding the body and helps to rebalance them. Light massage is also helpful. Deep tissue work needs to be avoided in highly sensitive people as it can trigger a detox response or a Herxheimer reaction. The emotional layers must be addressed. If someone can attain an expanded state, then healing is possible. You can't get better from these infections without a positive attitude. The more attention is directed to something, the more that something grows. If a lot of negativity is directed to a thing or issue, then it becomes more negative. Inversely, if positive energy is directed, it will shift the problem. Some people get these infections because it's their way to transcend whatever issues they have to work on in this lifetime.

Any kind of trauma can precipitate Lyme—rape, incest, molestation, a serious car accident, the death of

a significant person, physical abuse. It just needs to be
a severe trauma of any kind. Many have been beaten
up or abused in some way: either sexually abused,
physically abused, or verbally abused.

9: TREATMENT

LIKE MANY WITH CLD WHO have enough energy and endurance to venture out into their community, Cindy has become an advocate to help others to overcome these infections and get well. Her positive approach to life is stunning, as is her courage in facing her own illness.

CINDY'S STORY

Cindy recalls a tick bite when she was nine. She remembers being sick often throughout her life. But when she was 33 years old, symptoms began in earnest with flu-like symptoms and fever. Then came stiff neck and shoulders, headaches, and exhaustion. Creeping numbness and tingling followed. The headaches became constant and scared her enough to go to an urgent care clinic, where she was told it might be meningitis, but the tests were negative.

For over 10 years, providers told Cindy she had Multiple Sclerosis (MS), but Cindy didn't believe them. Then one morning, she felt the left side of her chin go numb. The numbness progressed, and she lost feeling in her throat and then the entire left side of her body. She was terrified. Numbness and tingling of her toes and feet followed next and progressed to her fingers and hands. Sharp pains, deep and low, in her abdomen occurred. Fatigue was overwhelming. Cindy would tear up when trying to communicate her symptoms to doctors, mostly because she could tell by the look on their faces that they didn't believe her. They would tell her, "I don't know what's wrong with you. You have too many symptoms." Test after test came up negative.

For Cindy, this time in her life was a mixed bag. She felt physically ill, but also extremely happy, as she had just met her future husband. She had never been happier. She knew, though, that something was wrong in her body. She saw multiple specialists and did numerous tests, all negative. The doctors were convinced "it was all in her head." Cindy was routinely offered antidepressants and anti-anxiety medicines, which she refused.

Marrying the love of her life, Cindy and her husband soon started a family. All three of the children were delivered C-section. With all her babies, she was unable to nurse as her pituitary gland wasn't working well. Being pregnant was great, but afterward, she felt unrelenting fatigue. It was shortly after the birth of her second child that Cindy came down with pneumonia for the first time. It took three months to get over it. Cindy had several episodes of pneumonia throughout the years after that. A few months after the birth of her third child, Cindy was so tired that she didn't want to leave her home. She feared socializing. Realizing this wasn't healthy, Cindy finally tried antidepressants, five different ones in a nine-week period. She would rock herself and curl into a fetal position and cry. Cindy couldn't get out of bed for weeks. She couldn't care for her children. Finally, a friend moved in with them to help.

A naturopath physician tested her brain neurotransmitters and found they were out of balance. So Cindy stopped the antidepressants and used natural amino acids that are precursors to neurotransmitters, and within a few weeks, she began to smile again. She felt alive and happy once more. However, her symptoms continued. She would be bedridden often. After 15 years of seeking help and a diagnosis, Cindy was told she had CLD. It was difficult for her to accept, as she had been tested repeatedly for Lyme and the tests were always negative. Finally, she was tested at Igenex lab by a Lyme-literate provider, and the results came back positive.

During the years before diagnosis, Cindy searched for the help she finally received. Besides the several bouts of pneumonia, she had root canals, was given cortisone injections into her spine for a supposed pinched nerve, and had her appendix removed unnecessarily. Remember that steroids like cortisone make treating Lyme more difficult.

Cindy has been dealing with brain fog for most of her adult life, another Lyme symptom. Once she got lost in her own laundry room. She found her phone in the refrigerator. She pays a nanny to help with the children and to drive them to school and activities so they are safe. She doesn't trust herself to take them places. Before the disease took a firm hold on her life, Cindy was active and loved to dance.

Cindy submitted over $100,000 in medical expenses to her insurance company and has paid over $20,000 out of pocket, excluding premiums and the cost of the nanny. Treatment is ongoing but some of the co-infections are gone. Cindy remains hopeful for complete recovery. She has a passion to help others who are suffering with these infections and to increase awareness so others do not have to experience what she has had to endure.

Treatment is a long process. It requires a lot of faith. It requires one to be compliant. A person has to be motivated and has to be willing to do the work that's required to get better; and when somebody's feeling sick and weak, it's hard to be motivated. Having someone to support and encourage is really helpful.

One of the things that happens when you start to treat is there's die-off of the "bugs," and in that process, a lot of dead cellular debris in the system that needs to be removed. The body has to be able to process this die-off and the neurotoxins that the bugs create. There are supplements, like zeolite and bentonite clay, and a medicine, a powder called cholestyramine, which is one of the original cholesterol medications that actually bind the die-off and toxins and remove them from the body. By taking a binder, you keep the body flushing, and by keeping the body flushed, then the body can better handle long-term antibiotic therapy.

There is a reaction that was coined back when treatment for Syphilis first began, called a Herxheimer reaction. It was Dr. Herxheimer who coined it. A Herxheimer reaction is one in which the symptoms a person is having actually get worse at the start of treatment. It has been shortened to a HERX response. If they had joint pain or they had nausea, those symptoms would worsen, and that would be called a Herxheimer reaction, and it meant that some of the bacteria were dying and the body wasn't processing the die-off well. People don't have these reactions if their body is clean and able to process and get rid of all of these substances.

People with long-term infection don't have clean bodies, so it's really critical to go slowly. One of my patients told me that another provider told her that her body was a cesspool that needed cleaning. For example, someone who's been really, really ill and reacts easily, and hasn't reached a place where they are able to process the die-off might be able to do only one drop of a tincture every three days, versus an optimal dose of 15 drops twice a day. They're so sensitive to the response that it makes them sicker. The immune system becomes so hypersensitive to this constant insult to it from these chronic infections that it goes haywire and reacts to everything.

What follows is a general overview of what might occur with treatment of CLD. It is not intended to be all inclusive. The current wisdom among many Lyme-literate providers is that antibiotics alone are not enough.

If you have had CLD for greater than a year, then it has adversely affected your immune system and your body's ability to detoxify and to eliminate the die-off of bugs and the neurotoxins they produce. IV antibiotics are an important tool if you have had CLD for longer than one year, if you are 60 years old or older, or if you have taken steroids and/or immune suppressants. For those with highly sensitive bodies that react to any small amount of die-off or toxin, then this can be a daunting decision.

IV antibiotics cross the blood-brain barrier more effectively getting at the bugs that are hiding in the brain. Many different co-infections respond to IV antibiotics, like Bartonella, Ehrlichia, Anaplasma, Mycoplasma, and C. pneumonia, as well as Borrelia or Lyme. IV antibiotics can be less devastating to the intestinal tract. The length of time necessary to do IV antibiotics ranges from three months to over a year. The medicines are usually pulsed, four days on and three days off. They are expensive, and it is rare that health insurance will pick up the cost, which is anywhere from three to four thousand dollars month. An indwelling central line or PICC line is indicated, and the cost to insert it is around fifteen hundred dollars—then there is the cost of maintaining the line.

Oral medications include antibiotics, antifungals, antimalarials, antivirals, and other medicines that deal with parasites. They are used in combination, depending on which infection is being treated. For example, when treating Babesia, it is necessary to use an antibiotic and antimalarial, and Artimisinin, an herb that drives the parasite out of the cells so the medicines can get them. Bartonella requires different antibiotics than Lyme or other bacterial co-infections.

While taking antibiotics, it is helpful to add the herbal tincture for the infection being treated. The tinctures are specific to each infection. Their benefits are supportive, and they do kill bugs. The bugs do not become resistant to them, unlike antibiotics, if it is necessary to stop due to a flare. The tinctures get in to the cells. The bugs can interfere with the energy pathways in the body, and the tinctures actually keep this from happening. They address the infections on all levels, unlike the antibiotics. Using antibiotics and tinctures together optimizes treatment. Finally, once treatment is done, the tinctures can be used for three to six months more to be sure all the bugs are gone.

Besides killing bugs, the immune system must be restored and detoxifying pathways cleared. This involves dietary change. It is important to create an alkaline environment as most people with CLD are highly acidic, and the bugs prefer an acidic environment. Increasing alkalinity is done with raw vegetable juicing, enzymes, and alkaline water. It involves eating more alkaline foods and less acidic foods. Fresh vegetables are alkaline. Beans, potatoes, and chocolate are acidic. Almonds are alkaline, and peanuts are acidic. Olive oil is best, and corn oil the most acidic. Red meat and shell fish are acidic, while wild game, fish, lamb and turkey are less so. Amaranth, millet, wild rice, and quinoa are alkaline. Other cereals are more acidic. Dairy is acidic. So the goal is to eat more of the alkaline foods and less of the acidic ones. Eliminating foods that increase inflammation is helpful, such as wheat, soy, and dairy.

Detoxifying principles include optimizing bowel health, using probiotics, fiber, colon cleansers, ensuring good hydration, minimizing toxic exposure, and optimizing cellular function. Probiotics are essential to help restore intestinal tract health. Approximately 75% of the immune system function resides in the intestinal tract or gut. Antibiotics and the bugs cause imbalance and the antibiotics kill beneficial bacteria, as well as the bad ones. The best probiotics contain multiple strains of Lactobacillus and Bifdobactrim bacteria and a beneficial yeast,

Saccromyces boulardii, that helps keep other unhealthy fungus or yeast from growing out of control. Without the probiotic, gastrointestinal symptoms worsen and fatigue increases. One of the best probiotics on the market is from Australia and is grown from human bacterial flora, so it colonizes the gut easier than others. It is called Progurt and can be purchased online.

Supportive nutrients and homeopathic medicines are available to upregualte the immune system. This is beneficial as it stops the hyper-reactivity to treatment that makes a sensitive person so ill. When the immune system response beings to function optimally, then it works with the treatment regimen to rid the body of infection.

Antioxidants support immune function and are free radical fighters. For example, glutathione, which is produced in the liver and is a potent antioxidant, becomes depleted by chronic infection. By using a liver supplement, glutathione production is enhanced. Liver inflammation can be controlled with Milk Thistle. Many of the medicines and some of the bugs can affect liver function and increase inflammation, causing a worsening of symptoms.

Magnesium, Co Q10, and L-carnitine support muscle function and any muscle benefits, including the heart muscle. Magnesium is sometimes helpful for decreasing cramping and easing constipation.

Some herbal remedies are amazing support for the liver, kidney, and lymph systems. When functioning optimally, these systems help rid the body of waste. It is possible to see liver and kidney lab values change using supportive therapies—and with no adverse side effects.

High grade, bioavailable multivitamin/minerals are very important. It is necessary to have a solid baseline of nutrients, so that it then becomes possible to add higher doses of specific nutrients, like Vitamin B12 or magnesium. Many nutrients require other nutrients to be present in order to work.

At integrative practices, it is possible to access IV supportive therapies. Examples include: amino acids to help rebuild tissue; high dose Vitamin C, B, and minerals; glutathione for liver support; chelation therapy to remove heavy metals; stem cell replacement to help rebuild the body; coloidal silver to combat infection of any kind; protocols to aid with detoxification; and more.

Hormonal abnormalities must be corrected to increase quality of life. Anyone with chronic illness has exhausted adrenals, which contributes to fatigue and energy levels. Adrenal glandular, along with herbal, support helps to rebuild the adrenals, which produce stress hormones like Cortisol. The adrenals are responsible for the circadian rhythm which affects our activity cycle. If imbalanced, not enough Cortisol in the morning makes it difficult to be active during the day. If too much Cortisol is produced at night, it is hard to sleep.

Thyroid imbalance is another concern, but easily corrected when treated. Optimal function contributes greatly to energy levels and metabolism. Sexual hormones are impacted, as well. Decreased libido is a common complaint. Women can suffer early menopause and irregular periods. Again, hormone replacement is available and helpful.

10: INANNA HOUSE

INANNA IS THE QUEEN OF Heaven and Earth and the Goddess of Love from the Sumerian Civilization that existed in 3000 BC in what is now known as Iraq.

As already mentioned in the first chapter, the current health care system is broken, and it is beyond repair. A new health care system is needed. The time is now. It is necessary to address all aspects of an individual—physical, emotional, energetic, mental, and spiritual—at the same time. There is not one way to accomplish this. Complexity demands that each individual be considered separately—*as an individual*.

In the current health care system, there is no place for the millions who are ill with CLD to get help when they are in need of more intensive support and care. No hospital exists that recognizes and treats these infections. For hyper-sensitive people, there is no place they can go to start IV antibiotics and get the needed hydration and IV medicine to control their symptoms while they react to the die-off and toxins. The costs for treating TBDs are staggering and insurance companies refuse to pay for them.

Every person that I have spoken with who is ill with CLD has mentioned their frustration that there is nowhere for them to go to get help when they are relapsing or herxing.

It is time for a change, a different way. It is time for a new paradigm for true health and healing. Inanna House will offer an oasis of peace, health, and healing.

Over 20 years ago, I was in Mexico on the Pacific coast of Oaxaca, floating in the water late one night, when I had a vision. I do not have visions very often, but this one was like a movie reel playing in my head, showing a place where people could come and receive the care needed to heal. I was aware that my vision was not unique—that many others would have a similar experience because it is so important and the world needs a new paradigm of health that truly serves everyone. For years, I held this vision. When my daughter was lying in the hospital, in agony, being undertreated and misdiagnosed, I realized that the time had come to create my vision. It became clear that this population of people with CLD desperately needed a place to go for help, where there would be competent care and treatment that would move them forward and help them to heal.

Inanna House will be a residence for debilitated, chronically-ill individuals—a place to receive supportive therapies in many modalities and to start treatment with IV antibiotics in a safe environment. The program is designed in one-week modules, although an extended stay beyond one week would be very common. It is a program designed to address all aspects of healing: physical, emotional, mental, spiritual and energetic.

I envision Inanna House resting on 10 to 15 acres in Sonoma County. There will be 24 private rooms with baths. It will be designed like a retreat center, with treatment rooms, a large meeting room for classes and

workshops, a steam room and infrared sauna, and
extra sleeping rooms for staff and residents who come
to learn. There will be a large 1 to 2 acre organic garden
that will feed the residents and provide food to a
separate, clean food restaurant on the campus that will
be open to the public. The grounds will include a pool
and hot baths. Gardens will surround the guest rooms.
Inanna House will truly be a place of peace, health, and
healing.

An endowment will be created in which people can
invest, so that those who have depleted their resources
can get help, too. Inanna House will not be able to use
any government or health insurance monies, because
then the government would be able to dictate what
could be done and what could not. It would be
unacceptable to limit my vision of what should be
possible. The intention is to blend all the best of what
health care has to offer, using various modalities in a
synergistic way to build and support, cleanse and
detoxify the body so that treatment of TBDs can be
maximally effective.

Some of the therapies planned include:

Using various modalities in a synergistic way to
build and support, cleanse and detoxify the body so
that treatment of TBDs can be maximally effective,
each week a resident would receive the following:

- IV therapy: this could include nutritional IV's
  with high doses of Vitamin C and B complex,
  minerals and trace minerals and amino acids;
  chelation to remove heavy metals, including
  lead and mercury; simple hydration for those
  who can't eat without vomiting; glutathione,

which supports the liver to function; and antibiotics as needed.

- Detoxification therapy for rebuilding the gastrointestinal tract, including Progurt, an intensely packed probiotic that is based from human flora that allows the intestinal tract to recolonize, and other probiotic support; and clearing the liver, lymph system, kidneys and gall bladder using neutraceutical and herbal therapies.

- Alkalinizing the body through diet. Alkalinizing the body eliminates the typical acidic environment in which bacteria, virus, and parasites thrive. This is accomplished with raw vegetable juices.

- Energetic therapies: This includes, but is not limited to, several modalities that help to support a balanced body, mind, and spirit. Included are:

  1. Cranio-Sacral Therapy, which is gentle work that allows the body to readjust by manipulating the Cranial Sacral System, which is a semi-closed hydraulic system contained within a tough waterproof membrane, the Dura Mater, which envelops the brain and the spinal cord. Dysfunction and ill-health can occur when pressure builds up in this system. With this therapy, the system is reset and balance can be achieved easier.

2. Frequency Specific Microcurrent uses low amperage targeted at specific tissues with specific frequencies for conditions like inflammation, fibrosis, scarring, pain, emotional issues, and many more. By directing the energy to specific areas in the body, the body is more able to rebalance and work toward healing www.frequencyspecific.com

3. Aromatherapy is used as an inhalant and a topical treatment, but also as an internal therapy for stimulating change and balance. For example, Laurel is used for the treatment of Lyme disease and makes an excellent topical oil as a repellent. Only the finest essences are utilized.

4. Sound healing is sound that stimulates different responses in the body and can be a powerful adjunct to other modalities.

5. Other possible therapies include LENS, which is excellent to release emotions that are impeding wellness, and Zyto, an energetic tool that picks up the energy of the problems a person is working with and then uses frequencies to correct them.

- Counseling to support the emotional shifts needed for healing, which include a process called EMDR that addresses any trauma that has occurred, including Post Traumatic Stress Disorder, abuse, rape, accidents, etc.

- Hormonal balancing: When someone has chronic illness, the hormonal system gets impacted severely. The adrenals become exhausted, and Cortisol levels eventually are so depleted that a person is significantly fatigued. Cortisol is the hormone that responds to any stressor, the fight or flight mechanism. When it is gone, so is the energy to live a functional life. The thyroid glands can become non-functional or depleted, as well as the sexual hormones. Without the balance of these hormones, life is truly difficult and without quality. Restoring these functions can be done with the use of natural hormones.

- Functional medicine support, herbal support, and treatment: Functional Medicine involves the use of neutraceuticals, rather than pharmaceuticals, for treating a problem. Many intestinal symptoms, including bloating, diarrhea, constipation, cramping, abdominal pain, and gas, become chronic and can lead to pain. Fatigue and loss of quality of life result. Bacteria and parasites are leading culprits. These can be treated once the problem is known through specialty testing. Having base line nutritional support is essential so that deficiencies can be addressed. Once the body is adequately supported, then healing can begin.

- Medical doctors, doctors of osteopath, naturopathic physicians, and nurse practitioners provide assessment and oversight and help with the individual plan for each resident.

- Infrared sauna and steam room treatment for circulation: Infrared Saunas are very supportive to a depleted body and help to restore vital energy. The heat also kills some of the bacteria.

- Light massage.

- Inanna House as clinical research center: Agreement to be involved in confidential, anonymized clinical research studies would be hard-wired into the treatment model. Inanna House will be a clinical research facility, as well as a teaching institution: a patient agrees to be a part of ongoing research and, in some instances, receive care from staffers-in-training when agreeing to be treated at Inanna House.

- Longitudinal patient follow-up studies: Inanna House tracks treatment success for years afterwards via detailed surveys to obtain valuable information to continuously improve and refine guest care, as well as data on possible relapses, reinfection, etc.

- Pioneering methods of environmentally-friendly tick eradication for Inanna House grounds and surrounding acreage to create a risk-free space for guest walks and recreation.

- Opening aspects of Inanna House healing programs (e.g. meditation/relaxation sessions) to non-resident, healthy persons who want some R&R and are willing to pay. This would help with funds to support Inanna House, as well as open the patient population to the energy of individuals who are not staff members or chronically ill, unconsciously helping to inspire patients with others who serve as energetic templates or reminders of life beyond TBD.

- Exploring parallels with the ancient Greek model for healing centers that treated the whole person—for example, having music therapy with live musicians.

Inanna House will be the first facility of many to model the new paradigm. It is part of the vision that Inanna House be built around the world. Many of these centers are needed as millions are in need of help.

ACKNOWLEDGEMENTS

I wish to thank Zoe Sexton for the support and encouragement she gave to me as I wrote this book. I could not have done it without her.

I also wish to give thanks to Neil Nathan, MD, and Eric Gordon, MD, of Gordon Medical Associates, for critiquing my work.

The people who shared their stories with me are courageous and amazing! I wish to thank them from my heart for allowing me to publish their stories. Some of their names are fictitious and others are genuine. I add their names with their permission.

ABOUT MARA WILLIAMS

NURSE PRACTITIONER AND ENERGETIC HEALER Mara Williams has been a health care provider for over 30 years. For 15 years, Mara worked in Hospice, helping people at the end of their life. For most of her life, she has been devoted to a spiritual practice and developing her gift of working with energy. This includes spending six months in Oaxaca State, Mexico, studying with a clairvoyant healer. Eventually, she returned to school at UCSF to earn a Masters and Certificate as a Nurse Practitioner so she could have a greater impact in helping people to heal. Currently, she specializes in treating people with Tick Borne diseases, using an integrative approach to help them attain greater health and well-being. The secret to healing is discovering the root cause of a problem, and this is what Mara does best.

Besides being a provider, Mara has personal experience as a mother of a child with Lyme disease. It has given her a greater understanding of what patients with TBD experience in the Medical World of Western Medicine and how difficult it is to find a Lyme-literate provider who recognizes and understands the complexity of these chronic diseases.

BIBLIOGRAPHY

THE INFORMATION PROVIDED ABOUT LYME disease, its incidence, and other facts were taken from lecture notes while attending workshops, from conversations with the providers I work with, and the websites of the California Lyme Disease Association and The International Lyme and Associated Disease Society.

I give credit to:

Eric Gordon, M.D.

Neil Nathan, M.D.

Wayne Anderson, N.D.

Azra MeEl, M.D.

Joe Burrascano Jr. M.D.

Ann Corson, M.D.

Steve Harris, M.D.

Richard Horowitz, M.D.

Byron White, Master Herbalist

REFERENCES

Buhner, S.H., *Healing Lyme*, Raven Press, Silver City, NM, 2005, pp 24-26.

Hay, Louise L., *You Can Heal Your Life*, Coleman Publishing, Farmingdale, NY, 1984, P16.

Kunz, Dora, *Spiritual Healing*, Quest Books, Wheaton, IL, 1995, foreword by Delores Krieger, p.1X.

RESOURCES

www.ILADS.org
Position papers and practice guidelines, diagnostic methods and treatments in the management of TBDs.

www.lymediseaseassociation.org
National patient advocacy organization.

www.turnthecorner.org

www.lymedisease.org
California Lyme Disease Association Information about TBDs.

www.lymeinfo.net
Medical literature summaries, legislative hearings transcripts, pending legislation.

www.columbia-lyme.org/index.html
Neuropsychological testing, medical workup, cognitive/neuropsychological problems.

www.igenex.com
Reference laboratory specializing in TBDs.

www.ncbi.nlm.nih.gov/entrez/query.fcgi
PubMed- Access to over 12 million Medline citations at the national Library of Medicine

Gordon Medical Associates
3471 Regional Parkway
Santa Rosa, CA 95403
www.gordonmedical.com